# Nursing Decentralization
## The El Camino Experience

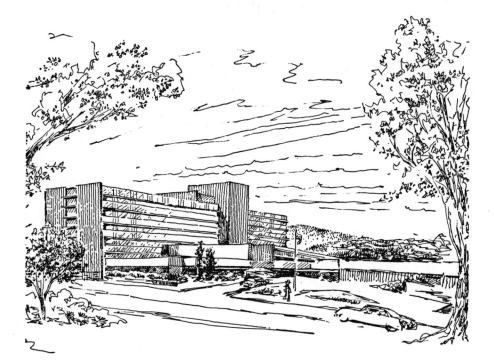

El Camino Hospital is a community-focused, 464-bed, general district hospital located on the San Francisco Peninsula. San Francisco is 35 miles to the
north and Santa Cruz 50 miles to the south. It is organized and licensed under
the laws of the State of California, and has full accreditation of the Joint
Commission of Accreditation of Hospitals. El Camino Hospital is affiliated
with DeAnza College in its Associate Degree Nursing Program and with San
Jose State University's Baccalaureate Nursing Program. Because the medical
staff is comprised of private physicians, opportunities exist for nursing
growth in a non-intern/resident setting.

# Nursing Decentralization
## The El Camino Experience

Joan Nietz Althaus, R.N., M.S.N.
Nancy McDonald Hardyck, R.N., B.A.
Patricia Blair Pierce, R.N., B.S.N.
Marilyn S. Rodgers, R.N., B.S.N.

*In conjunction with
El Camino Hospital
Nursing Service*

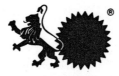

An Aspen Publication®
Aspen Systems Corporation
Rockville, Maryland
London
1981

*Library of Congress Cataloging in Publication Data*
Main entry under title:

Nursing decentralization: the El Camino experience

(Nursing dimensions administration series; v.2, no. 3)

Includes index.
1. Nursing service administration. 2. Hospital
wards—Administration. 3. Decentralization in
management. 4. El Camino Hospital. I. Althaus,
Joan Nietz. II. Series. [DNLM: 1. Nursing service,
Hospital—Organization and administration.    WI
NU587N v. 2, no. 3/WY 105 N0747]
RT102.N85    362.1'7    81-83018
ISBN 0-913654-76-0    AACR2

ISBN 0-913654-76-0

Manufactured in the United States of America


This volume was originally published by Nursing
Resources, Wakefield, Massachusetts and was included
in the Nursing Dimension Administration Series as Volume 2, Number 3.

# *Acknowledgments*

It is impossible to mention here all the people who helped in the preparation and typing of this book. We found every single person we approached to be willing to give of their individual time and talents, and we approached many! You out there know who you are—we couldn't have done it without you.

Carl Heintze was an untiring writer and special contributions were made by Nancy Smith, Gert Gillman, and John Fleming. Marlene Mayers has been our touchstone and anchor! Without her inspiration and practical assistance this book would never have been written.

Every person we have contacted in doing this book has encouraged and helped us. Thank you!

Joan Althaus
Nancy Hardyck
Pat Pierce
Marilyn Rodgers

# Contents

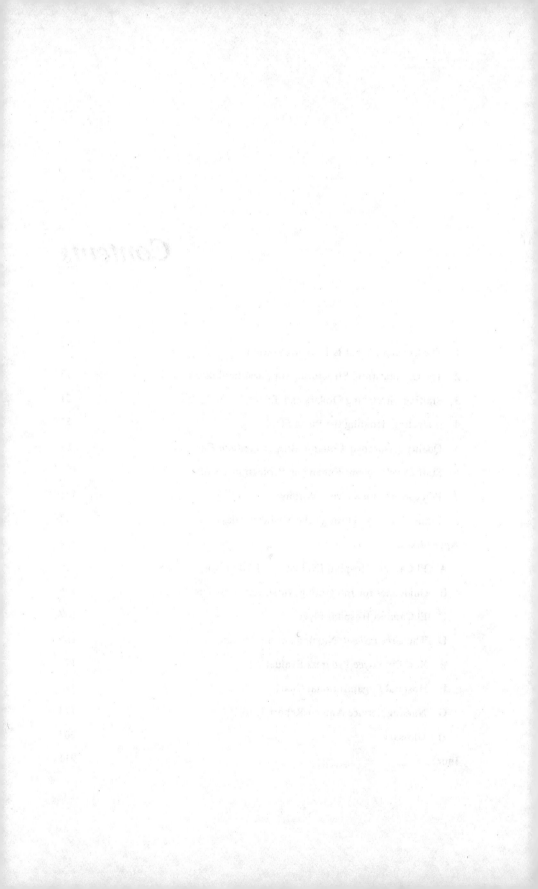

# *Preface*

The idea for this book originated with the realization that others were interested in the decentralized nursing organization structure at El Camino Hospital. Our story will be useful to those who care about a dynamic, humanistic, patient-centered nursing organization. We have found no references specific to nursing that completely describe a decentralized nursing organization in action. This book is our attempt to provide such a reference.

The book is divided into eight chapters, an appendix, and a glossary. Since decentralization is a relatively new concept in nursing, the first chapter contains an overview of our organization. The second chapter describes the operation of El Camino Hospital's decentralized nursing service. Chapters three through six provide detailed descriptions of the various components of the nursing organization at El Camino Hospital. Chapter seven summarizes our feelings and the results of our experiences with decentralization. Chapter eight is a fantasy trip into the future of nursing.

In writing this book, we have taken a very detailed look at ourselves and have documented more completely than ever before how our nursing organization functions. Hopefully this will be of assistance to the many people and agencies who have contacted El Camino Hospital for information about our organization. We know that all nursing services which become decentralized will be different. However they decide to progress, the information in this book may be helpful in deciding where to start and in being prepared for the changes that occur—changes both planned and unplanned.

# *Foreword*

Professionalism, autonomy, accountability, control, productivity, quality, employee satisfaction, and power are words that mean many things to many people. In the typical acute-care setting these terms have different meanings to staff nurses than they have to administration. How can a nursing service arrive at common definitions and then develop an organizational structure and processes that actualize these meanings? This book illustrates how one hospital's nursing service is doing just that.

This is a success story about decentralization. It tells about the ideals and values that provide philosophical guidance. It explains those more technical details of management that clarify how day-to-day operations are molded to reinforce and support the philosophy. It is an eloquent story of the commitment, struggle, joy, and pain that is inherent in developing an organization that truly supports professional care at the bedside.

Flattening and simplifying an organization's structure has many benefits for the professional practice of nursing. It places decision making with the person or persons most knowledgeable about care. It minimizes those many levels of hierarchy that often diffuse accountability and place the care giver at great distance from the focus of nursing practice decisions and authority. However, decentralization has its pitfalls. When an organization is flattened, the chief nursing administrator can end up with an enormous and potentially unwieldy span of control. Staff nurses find that they must be actively involved in making the policies that enable their practice. Involvement in all aspects of policy making adds an extra—but necessary—burden to the staff nurse's workload.

The usual methods of communication and decision making must be changed. The nursing administrator learns how to share power, how to participate as a peer yet be faithful to his or her sphere of responsibility. Head nurses learn how to be expert managers as well as clinicians. They learn how to foster both autonomy and cooperation in their staffs. They learn, too, how to share power and responsibility without violating their delegated arenas of accountability. Staff nurses learn how to function as professionals with ultimate answerability for patient care. Everyone's behavior and experience becomes more self-actualizing when decentralization is put into practice.

It is often said that nursing administrators must be able to deal with ambiguity. This is doubly true in a flattened organization. Disparate information comes directly from a multitude of sources. Many people and groups must be involved in every decision. It often seems to be a messy process. People do not quietly respond to directives. Instead, they react. Thus the administrator's life is not full of clean directives passed down the line; instead, it is full of negotiating, agreement seeking, and facilitating. Others in the organization find the same is true for them. The organization's life is filled with consensus reaching.

It is also filled with learning: understanding and using the technology of feedback mechanisms for budgeting, staffing, and quality; achieving skills in listening as well as talking; practicing honesty, clarity, and assertiveness; becoming more supportive and considerate; and learning how to problem-solve with both the macro and mini pictures in mind. Specifically designed educational programs are necessary to foster the learning needs of professionals in a decentralized setting.

Reading this book elicits many responses. There is incredulity over some of the practices that are described; delight in the philosophy and its results; concern about the possible unforeseen or long-term consequences of this kind of an organization; and ambivalence about the role of the nursing service administrator. It arouses enthusiasm and produces doubts. Most of all, it elicits a sense of hope for the future of nurses, nursing, and the well-being of its clients.

The four authors have worked as a committee, gaining information and insights from scores of people at El Camino Hospital. Typical of decentralization processes, this volume was commissioned by the Management Council of Nursing Service. Thus, although delegated to the committee of four, it represents a commitment by the entire nursing staff. The results of their efforts, as set forth in this book, represent a major contribution to the growing body of literature for the professionalization of nursing practice.

Marlene Mayers, R.N., M.S., F.A.A.N.

# 1

# The Concept:
# What is Decentralization?

We believe a revolution is moving through the nursing profession. Peaceful and progressive, this revolution evolves from within, and better patient care is its goal. The source of our unrest is that traditional hospital structure wherein authority and accountability are centered at the top of the nursing service. A growing number of today's nurses seek to replace this obsolete system with a new, decentralized organization in which the nurse at the patient's bedside is the key figure. Our revolution is dynamic: its principle contends that change is essential to vitality. At present, for want of a better term, we call our revolution *decentralized nursing.*

The search for ways to decentralize organizations is hardly new. What *is* new is the application of decentralization principles to nursing. From its beginning the nursing profession assumed a military structure, placing ultimate responsibility with top command and delegating direction and authority downward in a vertical hierarchy of importance. Too often, this autocratic organization found the patient at the very bottom, a kind of product handled on an assembly line by the nurse, just one of the workers. The fact that professional nursing evolved as a means of caring for the wounded in wartime undoubtedly had much bearing on its military modeling. Further, it was born in a time when the roles of males and females were clearly defined—some would say rigidly fixed—as master and servant rather than as equals. Under these dual shadows, nurses emerged as a group to be commanded rather than persuaded.

Early twentieth-century reformation of organized medicine only added to this rigidity. In organizing their ranks, doctors took for themselves a dominant role in the hospital. *They* directed; nurses *obeyed.* Most nurses were women, and the profession retained its subservient role.

Today all this is changing. In hospital after hospital, nurses are demanding a reformation of their own. To some degree this is a natural result of changing social and moral attitudes; the rise of feminism in the United States and the demand by women in all walks of life for status equal with that of men has certainly influenced the desire for structural change in organized nursing organizations. But in large measure these demands have sprung from the increasing concern among male as well as female nurses for improved patient care. Thoughtful nurses have realized that the patient should be paramount in the hospital nursing service rather than existing as a "product" that is handled at the lowest level of the nursing hierarchy. These nurses say the patient should be the focus of the entire nursing program. Moreover, the patient receives better treatment when considered as a whole person rather than a set of related—but often not integrated—tasks for the nurse.

Decentralization represents the merging of all these streams of change. The decentralization concept is rooted in the belief that the bedside nurse should have primary responsibility and authority for the care of a patient. Inherent in this principle is another: that nurses can be directed not from without but from *within.* Not all nursing outcomes are predictable. Nurses must have the flexibility and independence necessary to deal with changing conditions. Clearly, the realization of these themes cannot be achieved without a more *participatory system* of organization, a more democratic order of decision making.

## THE EL CAMINO CONCEPT

It is from these various cross-currents that we at El Camino Hospital have sought to build our system of decentralization. We believe our experience has been both unique and repeatable, one which in whole or in part can be adapted to other hospitals. In stating this, we do not mean to imply that the path to decentralization is necessarily easy. To create and sustain change is difficult, and we freely admit that our gains have not been accomplished without trauma. We have had to re-think many old methods and abandon some time-honored traditions. Decision making has not always been tidy or well organized, but it has been participatory. Many people have taken part in reaching our present level of organization.

Actively working together with supportive hospital administration, we at El Camino Hospital have developed what we believe is a working definition of decentralized nursing:

> *Decentralized nursing is a style of organization, communication, and decision making that fosters autonomy, accountability, and authority at the practitioner level.*

It is important to understand the many facets of this definition. This can best be done by examining each of its several parts individually.

---

**Exhibit 1-1.  The El Camino Hospital Nursing Service Organization**

---

## BEFORE DECENTRALIZATION

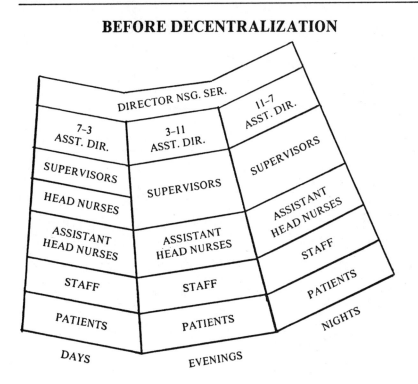

### Organization

The traditional system of nursing service organization (Exhibit 1-1) finds the director at the top of a pyramid, with various assistant directors, supervisors, and head nurses spread below, rather like the chicks beneath a hen's protecting feathers. Today at El Camino Hospital, that pyramid is reversed! Exhibit 1-2 tells the story. At the top of the triangle is the patient population for whom we care. Directly beneath we find the bedside practitioners who render that care; next come assistant head nurses, followed by head nurses. The Director of Nursing Service appears at the bottom.

The importance of this inverted pyramid cannot be overemphasized, for it means that the nursing service exists to support—not to draw upon—the patient. Indeed, the various levels of supervision beneath the bedside practitioner are now seen as support services, to assist rather than to impose their will on others. The inverted pyramid also implies increased emphasis on the role of the nurse at the patient's bedside. To this we have added the concept of

---

**Exhibit 1–2.    The El Camino Hospital Nursing Service Organization**

---

## AFTER DECENTRALIZATION

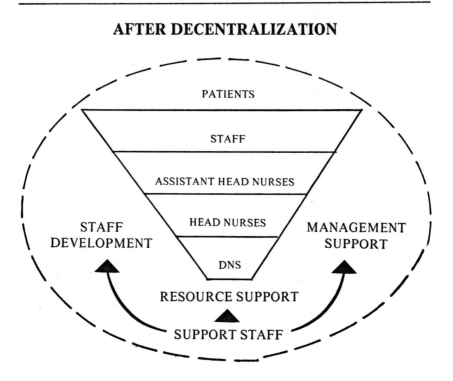

*primary nursing,* not a new idea but one that adapts uniquely to the decentralized nursing format.

We define primary nursing as a system in which each patient has a nurse who is responsible for his or her care. The primary nurse assesses a patient's needs and evaluates and plans for them. While on duty, she or he is responsible for the patient's care. Further, the primary nurse coordinates the nursing-care plan to be carried out by others when she or he is off duty. Such care is a 24-hour responsibility.

The nurse's role in the decentralized setting is like that of a primary-care physician outside the hospital. A colleagual relationship exists with the primary-care physician, and they work together at the bedside. The nurse is the initial resource available to the patient. Although nurses do not give all the care that patients receive in the hospital, they are responsible for it; that is, they delegate those services that they themselves cannot perform, and they have the authority to see that assigned tasks are carried out. From the rest of the nursing structure they draw the support and assistance needed to get the job done.

Just as this method centers attention on the patient, so does it focus on the bedside nurse as the most important part of the nursing process. It is a holistic view of the nurse–patient relationship. Rather than subdividing the nursing task into components parceled out to members of a team, one nurse works at the whole task of an individual's care. Thus the patient is seen as a human being rather than a technological assessment of needs.

### Communication

Decentralization of the nursing process cannot be successful without effective and continuing communication. In the traditional nursing structure, communication trickled down from the top and frequently became distorted in the process. In decentralization, nursing communication flows in all directions. It's genesis is what the staff nurse learns at the bedside. In some cases information may proceed directly from that nurse to the nursing director; but whatever route it travels, the emphasis in the process is on communication. There can be no responsiveness in a decentralized system unless there is communication. Much of the formal communication takes place in committees. Staff nurses from different clinical areas often meet together in formal settings with nurses from staff development and management support, and a new kind of colleagual communication occurs. One effective component of nursing communication at El Camino is our Nursing Service *Green Sheet,* a weekly newsletter printed on green stationery featuring timely information about new programs and personnel plus an update of ongoing activities. (A sample copy appears in the Appendix at the back of this book.)

While communication must travel vertically along the organizational structure to ensure support of nurses, it must move horizontally as well. If nurses are to arrange for continuing patient care when they are off-duty, they must be able to communicate their patients' needs to others at the same level within the system. Written care plans are essential to this function, but time must be allowed for verbal exchange as well. The feedback received from these other care givers is essential.

We can't overemphasize the importance of active feedback loops in all dimensions and levels. Effective communication cannot occur without the free exchange of information among all concerned parties. People who wish to make intelligent, best-possible decisions need all the information they can get. Without multidirectional feedback loops, decision makers will be operating without all available information. Of course, we all choose to ignore feedback at various times, but in the decentralized setting it is critical that the channels remain open. In formal meetings, contract setting, and evaluations, results are written and the feedback loop can be monitored. In committee meetings, the fact that all parties are represented ensures direct feedback among people with varied concerns; one person can hear directly from others how ideas are perceived. This leads to the achievement of compromise and understanding and the development of practical solutions acceptable to all.

A comprehensive computerized medical information system was developed at El Camino Hospital, and its presence has greatly enhanced nursing communication and documentation. Thanks to this system, nurses can spend more time at the patients' bedsides. It is with some reluctance, however, that we mention it at all in our discussion of nursing communication. While the computerized information has been enormously helpful to the El Camino staff, such a system is *not* an essential component to decentralization. The principles of decentralized nursing can be implemented with or without this convenience.

## Decision Making

To enhance both communication and decision making, we at El Camino view the organization of our nursing service as a participative, not an autocratic, process. This implies a kind of representative government, and involvement is encouraged. Nurses are urged to expand in the areas that interest them. These expansions may include committees, task forces, or projects at the unit or hospital level. When nursing policy is set by committee, membership takes on a new dimension. Sooner or later, staff nurses begin to realize that their working unit is being shaped by a group of peers in concert with a mixture of other line personnel—each with one vote. When a staff nurse tells a nursing committee of the need for a chemotherapy resource group, for example, she or he has the support and encouragement of peers. In addition, the nurse has their assistance in organizing the group and receives bureaucratic blessing on the final product. When this occurs, how can an individual feel powerless? More and more staff nurses recognize the value of committee participation as they discover it makes a real difference to them when decisions are made.

The management organization at El Camino Hospital is divided into two personnel categories. We call them *line* and *support.*

> *Line staff* are those personnel who have power and authority to act concerning patient care and to make either direct or management-type decisions in this regard. In our organization line personnel include the staff nurses, assistant head nurses, head nurses, and the director.

> *Support staff* are those personnel who provide line staff with expert advice, research, or information that enables them to function more effectively. Nursing coordinators provide management or administrative support; staff development instructors provide educational support; resource support people provide specialized services. Support staff assist line staff, who are the primary decision makers for the organization.

Under this arrangement, one major decision-making change finds head nurses assuming many of the responsibilities once executed by supervisors.

Nursing coordinators (formerly supervisors) are not line staff but support staff; that is, they are seen not as authoritarian, directing figures, but as support for unit personnel.

## Autonomy

Decentralization can be a large step toward professional autonomy within a bureaucracy. The concept of autonomy implies several things: Autonomous nurses have the authority to make their own decisions. Instead of constantly seeking permission or agreement from the next highest level of the hierarchy, they are able (and expected) to make most decisions concerning their patients. They become the focus of decision making, not the unwitting (and sometimes quite unwilling) vehicles of decisions made by someone else. They deal with patients on a one-to-one basis. To patients, an autonomous nurse means more than just another face that daily passes the bedside. She or he is *the* nurse not *a* nurse.

Delivery of nursing care is often a part-task system. When nursing is divided into its component tasks, the tendency is for a troop of faces to pass the patient daily. To the patient, and sometimes to the nurse, both the division of tasks and the multiplicity of faces is dehumanizing. Part-task nursing has other disadvantages: Part-tasks require only partial knowledge; those involved envision the whole as a team effort, an effort exerted by more than one individual. As in all technology, the tendency is to become proficient in a single task rather than to be versed in all that make up the entire function. The whole is neglected for its parts. One member of the team may be an excellent temperature taker but fail to appreciate the importance (or absence) of other vital signs.

We must add that when a task is broken into its components, it gets done only provided that everyone does their part; if components are missing, the task may never be completed. A team is only as strong as its weakest member. The team concept depends upon facing tasks that have predictable outcomes, and it works well when the pathways to completion are well trodden. It is far less successful when the reverse is true.

Inherent in the development of nursing as a whole-task system is the very real and vital factor of individual satisfaction. Autonomous nurses who care for whole patients, who minister to all their needs and see them through their hospital stays until the time of discharge, receive intangible but valuable rewards that the part-task team nurse seldom realizes.

As with any idea, the concept of autonomy has some disadvantages. Because the autonomous nurses need more knowledge to complete their tasks efficiently, their initial training periods may take longer and their need for continuing education never ends. The value of their work is individual, because individuals vary in performance, speed, skills, proficiency, and other qualities. Ongoing evaluation of the care given by the autonomous nurse may be more difficult simply because no two nurses approach the same problem in exactly the same way. Expected outcomes for good nursing care, however, remain unchanged.

A less obvious issue in autonomy is the traditional sexist socialization of female nurses against risk taking. Female nurses must learn to rise above the unconscious belief that they will be "unfeminine" if they take a stand. They must realize that assertiveness is okay, that they are indeed experts and at times more knowledgeable than physicians, head nurses, or other "power figures." When female nurses develop the self-esteem and sense of self-worth that they richly deserve, they will fall more naturally into autonomous roles. Until then, it will be a struggle.

It also is an open question as to whether or not autonomous, decentralized nursing is more cost effective than the traditional system. We believe it is, but we have only our own example from which to draw data. Nonetheless, it is certain that the more efficient a nurse is, the less costly she or he is likely to be. This very flexibility may facilitate cost savings.

## Accountability

A search through the nursing literature reveals a wide usage of the term *accountability,* but definitions of this term are sadly lacking. One article defines accountability as " . . . the responsibility for the services one provides or makes available" and " . . . a kind of accounting made of the productivity of an individual, group or institution."[1] We have found these definitions generally acceptable. If one is accountable, one is liable to be called to account for one's actions. The degree to which one is accountable depends upon the degree to which one has contracted to perform certain tasks. Thus it is intimately connected to whatever responsibility is assumed for actions or tasks. Just as the nurse is accountable to the patient, so is hospital administration accountable to the community from which our patients come.

Rarely does a collection of shared tasks foster accountability. There is good reason for this. The division of work tends to make no one responsible for anything or accountable for any mishap. To obtain high-quality nursing care it is necessary to focus both accountability and responsibility on the individual who is to perform the task.

Accountability is of increasing importance to the hospital nurse not only because of changes in legal liability, but also as a measure of the quality of care that a nurse or a nursing service renders. In the system of traditional nursing, most accountability rests on the nursing director. It diminishes as one travels down the nursing hierarchy and approaches the bedside. Accountability is most fragmented in the team-nursing/functional-nursing systems. Thus the nurse working as a part of the team is only partially responsible and accountable for the outcome of the team's efforts, even if there is an equal distribution of work. The "meds" nurse is accountable for medications, but cannot be expected to assume the responsibility for temperatures, especially if she or he has not taken them. Once medications have been dispensed, the team system relieves this nurse of further accountability.

In decentralized nursing, accountability centers on the nurse at the bedside. Therefore accountability and its handmaiden, responsibility, are necessarily individualized. It is the nurse at the bedside who is the repository of these two qualities; they rest neither with a team nor with the organizational structure of the nursing service.

We feel nurses are accountable when they are responsible and answerable to authority for their own actions. Accountability co-exists with autonomy.

## Authority

Clearly, no organization can operate without authority. Organizations that attempt to abolish it, no matter how noble their intentions, often succumb to anarchy. Yet, concentration of authority in the hands of a few seldom produces true cooperation. If cooperation is to be effective and continuing, some organization must be established. But cooperation tends to diminish in a ratio related to the size of any organization; the larger it becomes the less likely is true cooperation to take place. In large measure this is because cooperation depends on *communication,* and when communication becomes difficult, cooperative effort lags or ceases altogether.

To us this means that units within organizations must be limited in size. We can set no precise size limitation for effective function, but the units must be small enough to clearly define lines of accountability and authority. An organizational unit must be small enough to respond quickly to change, for it is a basic premise of the decentralized nursing system that change is ongoing. To this end, they are urged to work toward a consensus rather than wait for a decision from above. The head nurse of each hospital unit is the manager of that unit. There is a direct line of accountability between head nurses and the director of nursing. Throughout the structure of the organization, all units have available support in management, education, and special resources. Nurses are assigned to specific patients and they have the authority—as well as the responsibility—to provide the highest quality care for the patients under their supervision. When they begin their work at the hospital, nurses are specifically instructed that the basic tenet of the nursing service is that patients and their needs are primary to everyone's efforts. Our emphasis is on accepting responsibility for getting the job done, rather than telling others what should be done. The assumption of authority under this system cannot be made without an equal assumption of accountability.

## SUMMARY

We have attempted to clarify the concept of decentralized nursing by examining the six major points in its definition. All six are, of course, objectives. They have evolved through a half dozen years of experimentation and change from a traditional nursing system to decentralization. We freely admit that they represent a statement of philosophy, not a totally accomplished fact. Primary nursing care, for example, does not yet exist in all units of the hospital. It remains a goal toward which we are moving.

Staff nurses are not yet utilizing all the autonomy and power available to them. Their power can be acquired in several ways. The simplest is by just becoming familiar with the decentralized system. With increased understanding comes increased awareness of the total role of the staff nurse and the power that is inherent in his or her many responsibilities. As staff nurses become more familiar with what they can do professionally, they also become more familiar with their personal power: the ability to bring about changes through interaction with other individuals or with groups. In some ways, this is only a matter of recognizing that which they already have. However, the *willingness* of staff nurses to consciously exert this force is relatively new in nursing. The freedom found in decentralization makes it easy for this growth to occur. As nurses become more aware of their professional and personal abilities, they also become aware of many additional opportunities. These are often built into the decentralized system and are vested with power available to the nurse who will take it. Other evidence of personal power is found in the self-esteem and assertiveness that our staff nurses develop. This is advantageous when dealing with doctors, other departments, and peers.

If the use of power in the traditional nursing organization were examined, it would be evident that the people with power often do not have first-hand information or any personal interest in the situation being discussed. For example, traditional supervisors make staffing decisions, yet they have minimal knowledge of the patients on the units and the care necessary. They frequently wield power without sufficient information, and though the system is quick, it lacks credibility.

We have discovered that our way of functioning is not always a tidy process. The infighting which was now evident in a tightly controlled authoritarian nursing service is not in the open. It often seems that great amounts of time are spent in discussion of what is to be done before decisions are accomplished. But such discussions are representative; they do embody a consensus rather than a directive; they are participative. We believe that our concept is working.

Communication is sometimes simplified by the very complexity of the issues. When crucial problems must be resolved, the decisions are rarely a surprise because the people involved have had time to discuss and debate all sides of the problem. This depth of involvement makes it easy for the participants to communicate the decision to those who were not part of the decision-making process. Most important, the people who have the greatest need for the decision aren't forced to wait for it to filter down—they made it!

We have discovered that some tasks may take longer to complete than they did when they were specifically assigned. Working together has led to ideas, and ideas have led to cooperation and communication. In some cases ideas have proliferated so rapidly that they threatened to swamp the regular tasks. Yet we would not return to a system in which ideas were rare and born only from a few sources.

The change from centralization to decentralization has been gradual. Our "revolution" is really more of an *evolution,* and we believe it has provided us with a dynamic nursing structure. It is a structure that thrives on change; it is not static. Power has passed from nursing supervisors to head nurses. It is our ultimate goal that these portions which directly affect patient care continue to move to the staff nurses.

## REFERENCE

1.  Passos, Joyce Y., R.N., Ph.D. "Accountability: Myth or Mandate?" *The Journal of Nursing Administration,* May/June, 1973.

# 2

## *The Organization: Structuring For Accountability*

El Camino Hospital's new nursing organization is a simple one designed for decentralization. The task of moving to this system, where the nurse at the bedside is the focus of professional nursing care, has been largely accomplished, although some work remains to be done. In this chapter, we will describe the roles and responsibilities of individuals and groups within our decentralized organization.

A basic creed has been incorporated into the nursing-service organization manual:

- Our patients and their needs are central to all our efforts.
- The professional nurse must be free to use his or her knowledge to promote the patient's welfare and, in turn, must accept responsibility for the results of such judgment.
- The nursing organization must be structured so as to support nurses' accountability and autonomy.
- Expert teaching, coaching, advising, validating, and researching of care-related issues must be readily available in the form of expert management and resource personnel so as to continually maintain and improve effective care.

Our philosophy for change holds that decentralization of authority and responsibility is necessary; that all nurses are peers, no matter what their position in the hospital; that decisions should be gained from, and not imposed on, nurses; and, finally, that the nursing structure must be one that fosters and requires individual professional responsibility and participation.

The nursing service supports professional autonomy, requires individual accountability, and works to control and maintain a high standard of nursing practice. At the same time, it encourages greater participation in decision

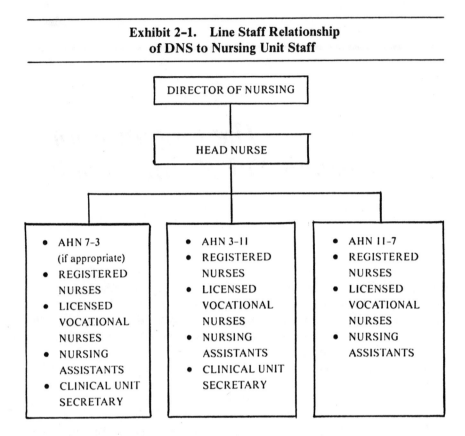

Exhibit 2-1.    Line Staff Relationship
of DNS to Nursing Unit Staff

making by all nurses and tries to simplify the levels of accountability within the hospital.

Line staff are people responsible for direct patient care and management—e.g., staff nurses and head nurses—as shown in Exhibit 2-1. Their organizational relationships appear in Exhibit 2-2, connected by solid lines to indicate line authority and responsibility. Resource support, management support, and complex members themselves are connected by dotted lines to indicate support roles. Line staff utilize the support staff and their own peers (whether in groups or singly) in making the important decisions that keep the hospital running. This concept is illustrated in Exhibit 2-3, which shows the top-heavy inverted triangle buttressed by support groups.

## INDIVIDUAL ROLES

### The Patients

As the inverted-pyramid structure implies, patients really *are* the most

**Exhibit 2–2.    Line and Support Staff
Nursing Service Organization**

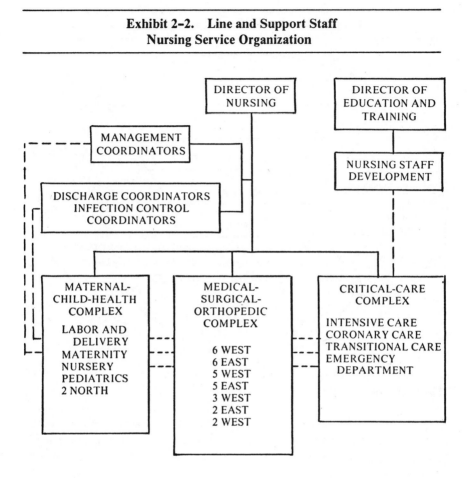

important part of our organization. This is evident in the type and quality of care they receive. From the time of admission, their personal preferences are identified and respected. The use of individualized care plans reflects this. As soon as patients are able, they are encouraged to assist in their own care. Thus they feel more in control of the situation while hospitalized and less lost or abandoned when they are discharged and must care for themselves.

But the decentralized system means more than that. It means that patients are closer to the other members of the organization. Not only may they talk with the quality assurance coordinator, they also may meet the staff development person or the shift coordinator. This interaction of patients, support staff, and staff nurses is very important in guaranteeing optimal care. Everyone has input and feedback about what the patient wants as well as what the patient needs.

---

**Exhibit 2–3.    Nursing Service Organization**

---

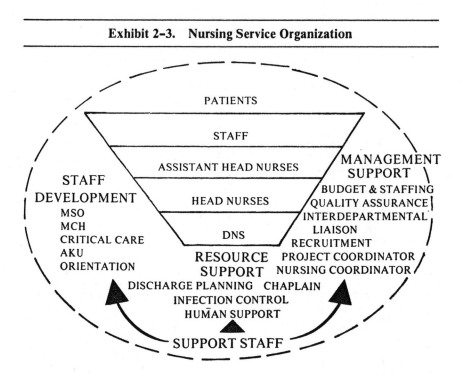

### The Staff Nurse

In a decentralized nursing system the staff nurse is the direct care giver. It is on this essential premise that the entire system is based. The eventual goal at El Camino Hospital is for all nurses to become primary-care nurses. By this we mean the following:

- One-to-one nurse–patient relationships.
- Patient-care decisions made by the primary nurses.
- Clear allocation of authority and accountability for nursing decisions.
- Twenty-four-hour accountability for care-planning for assigned patients.
- The care planner is the care giver.
- Direct communication from care giver to care giver, physician, and/or other health disciplines interacting with the patient, and vice versa.
- Inclusion of the patient in the planning of his or her care.

The emphasis of the El Camino nursing service is toward primary-care nursing, which focuses on the nurse at the bedside as the center of the organization's plans and operations. Ideally, this means that nurses operate as independent practitioners with their own autonomy, authority, and accountability. Their ability to function in this role ensures continuity of care and provides them with personal satisfaction. They have a 24-hour responsibility for their patients, but they receive a 24-hour satisfaction from their work. They maintain a one-to-one relationship with their patients, and provide the key to decentralized decision making about those patients. Primary-care nursing means clear allocation and delegation of authority and accountability for nursing decisions.

Currently, in most nursing units at El Camino Hospital, the total conversion to primary care remains incomplete. But we are working towards the day when all staff nurses will be primary nurses, individually assuming full nursing responsibility for their own patients.

**The Assistant Head Nurse**

The role of the assistant head nurse is to maintain the 24-hour continuity of leadership in the absence of the head nurse and to assist the head nurse in the clinical unit management. The assistant head nurse also helps create and maintain an environment conducive to growth and learning among the staff.

Job functions of the assistant head nurse include coaching of personnel, staffing and scheduling, plus monitoring of acuities and productivity for the shift. They are responsible for the quality assurance aspects of patient care: reviewing care plans, communicating audit results, and assisting in the formulation of any necessary remedial actions.

Public relations is an important role of the assistant head nurse. She or he is responsible for communicating and problem solving with the other departments, consulting with peers in committee meetings, and interacting as necessary with patients' families. The assistant head nurse participates in counseling and interviewing sessions, and provides personal as well as professional support and stimulation to the Head Nurse.

**The Head Nurse**

The Head Nurse is the department head of a unit, and in this capacity assumes a 24-hour responsibility for that unit. Head nurses report to the Director of Nursing Services, and their staff nurses report to them.

Head nurses organize their own units. They delegate responsibilities within the limits of their contract with the Director of Nursing Services and within the guidelines and legal policies of the hospital. They are responsible for the hiring and termination of nurses within their units. Head nurses also provide counseling, job clarification, assessment of general patient needs, and budget preparation; they obtain inservice education (staff development) for the staff and offer management support for assistant head nurses.

The head nurse functions as a patient advocate, intervenes in crises, and supports families. She or he serves as a support and resource person for the nurses within the unit. As a role model, the head nurse also takes part in direct patient care. Clearly, clinical excellence is something the head nurse seeks to instill in all members of the staff; in addition, personal involvement in clinical care facilitates a better understanding of the patient's concerns and provides a constant reminder that the patient is the consumer of nursing service.

## The Director of Nursing

The director of nursing is the chief executive officer of nursing services. This individual is accountable to the hospital administrator and board of directors for maintaining the quality of nursing care. Today, the duties of this position are different from those of the earlier, traditional organization. Continuing responsibilities include supervision of budgeting, staffing, and evaluation. Also, the director still acts as nursing spokesperson with hospital physicians and administration. Now, however, there is a much greater emphasis on increasing support and rapport between nursing groups and on guiding and coordinating the entire organization in assuming responsibility for its own decision-making processes. As we see the director now, she or he directs, influences, guides, and coordinates.

The director carries out these complex responsibilities through a variety of formal and informal relationships with the rest of the nursing staff. She or he meets with head nurses at least once a month. The same schedule of meetings is maintained with the management-support section and with the director of education and training. All members of the nursing staff may confer with the director on a one-to-one basis as required or desired. While no strict schedule for such meetings is maintained, this is possible because the director of nursing services maintains an "open-door" policy and makes an effort to be available to all staff members. Because the director may also serve with staff nurses on committees and task forces, the nature of his or her relationships varies from formal accountability interchange to informal peer relationship and participation.

The director of nursing services no longer functions with assistant directors or supervisors. Indeed, line authority leads directly to the head nurses. This authority continues from head nurses to assistant head nurses, staff nurses, licensed vocational nurses (LVNs and LPNs), nursing assistants, orderlies, technicians, and unit secretaries.

Head nurses and coordinators who are accountable to the director set management objectives that provide the criteria for their performance evaluations. These objectives are defined and the priority is given to objectives which bear on the quality of patient care, staff satisfaction, staff development, and labor productivity. It is the duty of the director to review performance and initiate action wherever results do not meet objectives. The director of nursing services also meets with nurse representatives of departments separate from nursing service for coordination and support. These units, which have separate directors, are the operating room (including the recovery room and the ambulatory surgery center), the artificial kidney unit (AKU), and the psychiatric unit.

## GROUPING FOR EFFICIENCY AND SUPPORT

### Complexes

Complexes are made up of several similar or related nursing units. They correspond to the traditional wards or floors found in most hospitals. The three El Camino complexes are Maternal-Child-Health (MCH), Critical Care (CC), and Medical-Surgical-Orthopedic (MSO). The five Maternal-Child-Health units are labor and delivery, maternity, nursery, pediatrics, and gynecology. Critical Care has four units: intensive care, coronary care, transitional care, and emergency. The Medical-Surgical-Orthopedic complex is made up seven units: two medical, two surgical, one orthopedic, one short-term surgical, and one that is a combination of genitourinary, renal, and orthopedic. The management and resource support and staff development sections provide assistance for the complexes.

The head nurses in each complex meet for purposes of team management, mutual problem solving, decision making, goal development, information sharing, and feedback. The team building that results from these activities is crucial to the effective management of a decentralized organization. Each complex rotates its leadership so that head nurses take turns as complex captains, sharing in responsibilities and influence. The complex captain sets the agenda for the meetings and contacts support personnel to attend as necessary. Chapter 3 will define further the role of complex captain. The director also meets monthly with each group of head nurses.

### Management Support Group

The management support group is responsible to the director of nursing services. There are two full-time and three three-fifths time shift coordinators for administrative and staff support on the 3–11 and 11–7 shifts. On days, there are three full-time coordinators, one each for budget and staffing, nurse recruitment, and quality assurance. There is an additional four-fifths time position (days) for interdepartmental liaison. Periodically, a special-projects coordinator (days) is chosen to work with the management support group.

Nursing coordinators can be delegated authority for decision making by the head nurses, the director of nursing services, and hospital administration.

Coordinators utilize meetings to get work done and to maintain personal contact with head nurses, assistant head nurses, the director of nursing services, and the staff development instructors. They also may attend other necessary meetings, such as those of the nursing management council and the medical staff. The position requires management skills: ability to work well with people and to problem solve at the administrative level. At least one nursing coordinator is available on each shift to handle day-to-day nursing-service problems. On day shift this trouble shooting is handled by rotating "officer of the day" duty among the coordinators. Evening and night shifts usually find only one coordinator on duty.

The nursing coordinator for budget and staffing is a resource and support person for head nurses and their assistants. This individual is involved in the budget process and helps ensure coordination and completion of budget goals within the nursing service. The budget and staffing coordinator also supervises the staffing clerks and assists head nurses in solving short-term staffing imbalances.

As you may have guessed, the coordinator for nurse recruitment recruits nurses. This involves close communication with head nurses to determine qualities, skills, and experience desired in a new employee. The recruitment coordinator conducts prescreening and initial interviews for all nursing personnel, and is also available as a resource on employee relations and labor law for individuals or groups.

The nursing coordinator for quality assurance collects the data regarding quality of nursing care and aids in setting standards for the maintenance of its excellence. This person assists in developing patient-care standards, provides methods of evaluating them, and acts as a resource for refining the auditing processes.

Coordinator for interdepartmental liaison is a position unique to our decentralized organization. It provides an avenue of communication that links all other departments with nursing, eliminating for these departments the difficulty of trying to communicate with 16 different head nurses. The coordinator assists in the development of mutual interdepartmental policies and programs. A primary objective of this role is the type of intervention that will free head nurses from lengthy problem-solving sessions with support service departments. The coordinator for interdepartmental liaison also collaboratively updates and monitors nursing departmental policies.

A special-project-coordinator is chosen periodically from among the head nurses by the director of nursing services. This nurse will serve for three or four months for the purpose of researching two or three identified issues or projects, such as the clarification of complex-captain roles, head-nurse orientation, lateral promotion, or preparation of the annual report (see Appendix). The choice of a special-projects coordinator is based on an individual head nurse's experience and interest in the particular projects; later the head nurse returns to his or her previous position.

The special-projects coordinator works very closely with the director of nursing services and the other nursing coordinators. The interlude provides an opportunity to view the organization from their perspectives. This coordinator is expected to assume the duties of the director if he or she is absent, and to fill in for the director at meetings or community functions.

Such a change in environment can be a welcome sabbatical from the many pressures of the head-nurse position. The unit he or she leaves behind is taken over temporarily by a nurse designated as the acting head nurse. Thus someone else's horizon is broadened, new experiences are made available, and new perspectives are gained. This multifaceted job enrichment serves the organization and the people well, besides being a creative way to accomplish special projects.

The shift nursing coordinators (3–11 and 11–7) are key support persons to the staff on those shifts, to the head nurses, and to the hospital administrators. They have primary management accountability in the absence of the hospital administrator and are called upon from all hospital departments to interpret or enforce hospital policy. Their role is also clinical in nature, and they act as a resource for nursing units with patient-oriented problems. They support and coach assistant head nurses and staff in crisis situations, problem identification, and problem solving. They are knowledgeable in staffing and budgeting, which enables them to support and coach in the areas of staff utilization, patient acuities, and unit productivity. They foster the concept of decentralization by maintaining their consultant role. The coordinators are always available to encourage and support staff nurses responsible for making decisions on their respective units. However, they refrain from making the decisions themselves.

## Resource Support

The discharge planning coordinators and the infection-control coordinator are two more major staff support positions that are directly responsible to the director. The two full-time discharge planners assist the nursing staff, patients, and patients' families with post-hospitalization needs, assessment, and care of the patient. They are very knowledgeable about community resources available to patients, and they work very closely with the Department of Social Services and the skilled nursing facilities.

Infection control has one full-time nursing coordinator who acts as a resource on all infection-control issues. This individual provides consultation and inservices as necessary regarding isolation procedures and aseptic techniques, and is responsible for the surveillance of community and hospital-acquired infections. Relevant statistical summaries and reports prepared by the infection-control coordinator are sent to local and federal agencies.

The chaplain works with volunteers to meet the spiritual requests of the hospital patients and staff.

The human support group is a multidisciplinary team that includes a family therapist, a registered nurse, a psychologist, and many trained volunteers. Services, consultation, and training are offered in areas of stress reduction, emotional support, crisis intervention, and grief therapy. Trained volunteers provide respite care and bereavement follow-up to patients and families dealing with life threatening or terminal illness. All human support services are available to hospital staff, physicians, and community members as well as to patients and their families.

## Staff Development Group

The staff development group's primary responsibility is for education as it bears on nursing practice. This group is also responsible for a number of other tasks including the orientation of new employees, research into better methods of nursing education, health-career counseling, and continuing education for staff members. The group supports and encourages commitment on the part of the nursing staff to high nursing-care standards through a variety of educational means. It is also concerned with community and patient education and is responsible for hospitalwide management and organizational development programs. The staff development group is responsible to the director of education and training.

Each support group plays its part in the effort to improve all communication within the nursing service. Although they are responsible to different department heads, they work together and with other hospital personnel. This effort is centered on the belief that nurses should see the nursing service as *participative.* Equality of communication and decision making is necessary to create individual responsibility and accountability.

## FORMAL COMMUNICATION AND GROUP DECISION MAKING

Much of the working organization's formal communication takes place in committees. For decentralization to be effective, staff-nurse participation in these committees is vital, and careful attention is given to encouraging a good cross-section of nursing representation. The input of staff nurses from different complexes and shifts, staff development, and management support is needed whenever the subject matter is relevant to their jobs. Staff nurses at times feel intimidated by their head nurses and support personnel, many of whom were their supervisors under the former organization. To overcome this psychological barrier, head nurses and support people often remain in the minority, thus minimizing any "advantage" they may exercise over staff nurses. Meeting times are set by the group so that the hour is convenient for all. As staff nurses gain confidence in relating to support nurses and head nurses on a peer level, their self-esteem increases and a sense of autonomy sets in. Stereotyping and misconceptions diminish, and facts replace rumors.

Nursing committees make more relevant and practical decisions as a result of staff-nurse input. Staff nurses learn of the latest developments within the organization, and committee work often gives them a broader perspective. As staff nurses voice their concerns or make suggestions regarding a topic or issue, they become increasingly aware of their value as professionals and direct care givers. Their investment in a committee's work or decision leads to greater effectiveness in taking it back to their respective nursing unit and assisting in the necessary implementation.

Another part of the formal communication system is the *Green Sheet,* our nursing service newsletter. It is read by all nursing personnel and contains such items as (1) meeting times and places (with agendas if appropriate); (2) any information and announcements of specific interest to staff nurses—e.g., new product information, policies, reminders; and (3) current career opportunities. In agreement with the hospital's philosophy to promote from within whenever possible, and in keeping with the concept of increased autonomy for staff nurses in all phases of their jobs, all available nursing positions (or any positions which might best be filled by nurses) are advertised. This gives staff nurses equal opportunities to apply for positions that interest them. It also gives the department seeking a new employee the best possible pool from which to select. Only if it is determined these positions cannot be filled from within is outside advertising initiated.

This system of filling positions has replaced the informal grapevine approach to job placement within nursing. It is a definite improvement over the old system, where people in power made their selections without ever announcing that the position was open. Depending on the level of the position, the selection process may vary from a personal interview to interviews by a panel. Staff nurses give input on applicants for positions on their units, including that of head nurse. Likewise, head nurses are involved in selection of support and line personnel, including the director of nursing services. Advertising open positions is one of the most vital elements of the *Green Sheet* and probably accounts for much of its wide readership.

There are several standing committees that have hospitalwide application. These are Management Council, Executive Committee, Nurse Practice Committee, Nursing Care-Planning Committee, Product Evaluation Committee, and MIS (Medical Information System) Nursing Committee. Time served by staff nurses on these committees is compensated, usually by the use of the head nurse's AD (administrative) time allocation.

**Management Council**

The Management Council is the decision-making body of nursing service.

**Exhibit 2-4.    Lines of Communication and Decision Making**

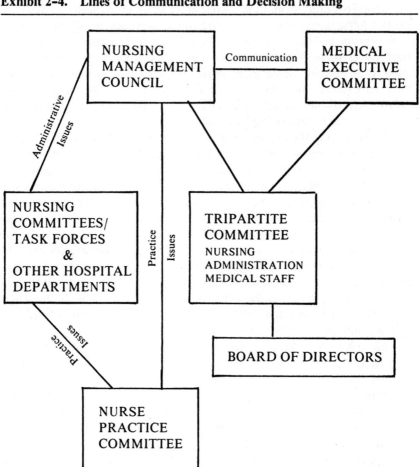

Decisions are subject to approval by the nursing director. Voting members, who are chosen by the group they represent, include all head nurses, one staff nurse representative, two management support representatives, one staff development representative, as well as the director of nursing. Other support personnel are encouraged to attend. Its agenda is published one week in advance of its monthly meeting in the *Green Sheet*. Issues such as the new float policy and the nursing dress code were discussed and obtained approval here. All policy recommendations from any of the other nursing committees must be approved by Management Council before becoming "official."

The agenda for Management Council comes from many sources. All nursing committees bring policy questions and issues to Management Council for final consideration. Practice issues must always come via Nurse Practice Committee. Administrative issues can come directly from any group or individual to Management Council. (See Exhibit 2–4.)

Staff nurses may make presentations in the role of representatives of committees or interests. Other agenda items may include such things as infection control or CPR statistics, and students asking assistance or support for research projects or relaying results of such work. Anything that needs official nursing sanction, communication, or information sharing can be brought to this group. Meetings last no longer than two hours; if issues require longer discussions, special meetings are called or further work is delegated to a task force.

Because consensus is necessary, decisions frequently come only after lengthy and complex debate. Some issues may be thorny and painful, but when the vote is taken and a decision reached, the blame or credit belongs only to us, not "them."

### Executive Committee

One of the major standing committees is Executive Committee. Its primary function is to enhance participative management decision making and communication flow. This committee meets with the director to review issues and make recommendations which are then discussed and resolved by the Management Council. It is also a task-oriented group that sets and accomplishes tangible goals during its tenure.

This body includes representation from all three shifts and all job categories within the nursing service. Representation is unique. Membership is as follows:

- Four staff nurses or assistant head nurses: one from Critical Care, one from the MCH complex, and two from MSO.
- Four head nurses: one from Critical Care, one from the MCH complex, and two from MSO.
- One management support group representative.
- One staff development representative.
- One float nurse.
- One licensed vocational nurse.
- One nursing assistant.
- One clinical unit secretary.

Representatives attain Executive Committee membership from a variety of intradepartmental methods. Some are appointed or chosen by peers, others by virtue of their position. All meetings are open forums and anyone interested is invited to attend, either as an observer or to request time on the agenda. Committee membership is limited to three months, and the meetings of the committee are announced in advance in the *Green Sheet.*

At the first meeting, the group brainstorms various project topics that could be accomplished in a three-month period. The topics are prioritized and the committee agrees on one project. One idea generated from the Executive Committee was establishing an annual staff meeting. It is a social as well as professional occasion. All active nursing committees display their activities and accomplishments in booths, and refreshments are served. Communication has been greatly enhanced as a result of this function. Another recent Executive Committee idea was to request "helpful hints" from staff nurses in patient care: a sharing of ideas and methods that nurses have found helpful in their daily work. These are printed periodically in The Green Sheet with contributors' names and nursing units.

Other projects undertaken by past Executive Committees have included establishing a float policy, revising the nursing dress code, sponsoring an open house to assist in recruitment, and assisting night staff by keeping the cafeteria open at night.

## Nurse Practice Committee

The function of the Nurse Practice Committee is to review, research, and make recommendations regarding issues that affect the delivery of quality nursing services. This process usually results in development of nursing procedures and protocols or referral to the Tripartite Committee (see Exhibit 2-4) for standardized procedures. The Tripartite Committee is a group comprised of an administrator, the Director of Nursing Services, and the Chief of Medical Staff that provides joint input for developing standardized procedures as defined in the California Nurse Practice Act of 1974.

The Nurse Practice Committee meets monthly and the membership is comprised of a staff nurse from each nursing unit. Evening and night shifts are represented. There is also a head nurse from each complex, a staff development representative from each complex, the director of education and training, the director of nursing service, a management support representative, the audit coordinator, and the coordinators responsible for procedure and policy. Membership is for one year. Nurses chosen to serve are acknowledged by their peers to be outstanding clinicians, generally well read and informed about their area of practice. An assertive, professional style as well as analytical skills in issue identification and problem solving are important qualifications for appointment to this committee. The Nurse Practice Committee was formed in 1977 subsequent to the passing of the California Nurse Practice Act. Its stated mission is (1) to stimulate an awareness of personal beliefs about nursing practice at El Camino Hospital and to communicate those beliefs to others; (2) to define standards that facilitate quality care utilizing nurses as collaborative members of the health care team; (3) to define, strengthen, and enhance both the humanistic and the technical areas of nursing practice; and (4) to identify and propose ways in which nursing can creatively fulfill the needs of the community with consideration of existing resources and constraints.

The accomplishments of this relatively young committee have been numerous. Policies and procedures have been researched, developed, and communicated. Nurses, physicians, and administration have been oriented to the role, functions, and achievements of the committee, as well as to the California Nurse Practice Act itself. Most important, however, is the meeting together of nurses to discuss, research, and pay attention to nursing practice issues as they continue to carry out the original (and current) mission. A copy of a Nurse Practice Committee flyer appears in the Appendix of this book.

## Nursing Care-Planning Committee

The Nursing Care-Planning Committee is made up of staff nurses—one from each unit in the hospital. There are also representatives from staff development, quality assurance, the head nurse group, and the computerized medical information system (MIS). (The basic care planning system for the hospital is handled by MIS, so any changes must be coordinated by that department.)

The purpose of this committee, which usually meets twice a month, is to monitor care planning at El Camino Hospital. The nurses who serve on it are care-planning enthusiasts. They are molding the care-planning system into a practical tool with which to communicate, document, and audit the quality of nursing care. These staff nurses act as care-planning resources on their respective units and work with the head nurse to improve and increase the use of care planning. They are often involved in gathering data about the status and use of care planning on their units. This committee is critical to keeping the care-planning system current and practical.

## Product Evaluation Committee

The purpose of this committee is to evaluate new products, to monitor the usage of nursing supplies with emphasis on quality of care and cost containment, and to review and evaluate on a regular basis all high-volume, high-price items.

The Product Evaluation Committee is composed of one staff nurse representative from a medical unit, a surgical unit, an orthopedic unit, the intensive-care unit, and the emergency department. Further nursing representation on the committee includes staff development, operating room, management support, and infection control. Representatives from other departments include the purchasing agent, materials manager, a biomedical engineer, the manager of central distribution, and a management engineer.

The committee meets monthly and devotes one meeting a year to a brainstorming session geared toward product development.

This committee reviews new products for quality, effectiveness, workmanship, convenience, and durability. Product safety and cleanability are also taken into consideration. It has been found that those nurses using the products have the expert knowledge necessary to make quality, cost-effective decisions.

### MIS Nursing Committee

The MIS Nursing Committee is still another example of nurses becoming involved in the decision making that affects their everyday working life. The committee is chaired by the Quality Assurance Coordinator and includes PM assistant head nurses from all units, and representatives of the computerized medical information system known at El Camino as MIS.

Since the MIS is an integral part of nursing at El Camino, it is important it remain as trouble-free and up-to-date as possible. This group reports and documents problems and participates in the development of creative solutions. They provide suggestions for future MIS developments and are a valuable communication link between the MIS representatives and the nursing units. It is especially convenient that they interface with both night and day shift, providing a perspective that is not always evident to day-shift workers.

The committee minutes include a "process list" which lists all problems reported, who is responsible for the solution process, and which step the process is in each month. This list has been especially useful for tracking activity and showing progress (or lack of it). It prevents the "loss" of problems that should be taken care of and shows when a solution has been implemented. The concept of utilizing those nurses close to the bedside for decision making is the major emphasis of this unique type of committee. No matter *what* the issue, nurses who are close to it should be involved in the decisions.

### Other Groups

Other committees and task forces meet to develop special projects or for a certain purpose and may disband when the project or purpose is accomplished. Membership in these groups is determined by who is most knowledgeable and most closely affected by the subject in question.

### INFORMAL COMMUNICATION

Informal communication loops exist at and across all levels and are multifaceted and infinite throughout the organization.

The most obvious such loop in the nursing structure is that involving the nurse and the patient. Nurses should be in constant communication with their patients, receiving and sending messages about their care. This particular loop did not always exist in traditional nursing care; it was frequently a one-directional line from nurse to patient. With its development, patients participate actively in decisions about their own care. The Quality Assurance Coordinator monitors this loop by patient interviews to assess the patient's condition, perceptions, and desires, comparing them with the nursing care plan and nurse's perceptions.

Similar kinds of loops exist at other points in the nursing service. One of these is the communication between the staff nurse and the head nurse. Another is between the head nurse and the director of nursing service. Still others exist between the management support or staff development groups of the nursing service and those units that provide direct patient care. Other lines cross and recross from person to person in ways stranger than fiction! In each case, loops of communication are possible and encouraged. With multidirectional communication it is possible for a wide array of necessary feedback to be developed and maintained.

Although initial problem solving rests on their shoulders, the staff nurses have considerable assistance available. Besides the equipment, skills, and teamwork on their own units, they can call upon the staff development and management support groups for help. It is important that they be aware of the array of resources available for use at their discretion.

## CONTRACTS

Still another way of communicating is through contracts. Contracts are agreements between individuals—or, in some cases, between units or groups of individuals. They concern mutual goals or expectations and how they are to be accomplished.

Contracts may be either written or oral, but usually they are formalized in writing. The basic elements of a contract are a set of conditions, a time frame for the beginning and completion of each task, and the names of those involved or responsible for tasks. The use of a contract is considered a more binding method of communication than a simple verbal agreement because it enhances clarity, and it may also be used as a way of evaluating the performance of those individuals named in the contract.

Contracts have the advantage of refining and clarifying objectives and methods of achieving work. Obviously not all tasks require contracts, but contracts do function as a way of pinpointing the expectations and responsibility for what is to be done. They also communicate more clearly how, when, and by whom tasks are to be completed and thus are an important element in the development of accountability in the decentralized nursing structure.

These stated goals and objectives are built-in monitors to ensure completion of the communication feedback loop to both contractees. At the end of the agreed time it can be readily identified whether or not the stated goals have been accomplished.

In decentralization, organizational goals are developed by the director of nursing services with input from other members of the organization. The nursing organization is represented in this process by the nursing coordinators, staff development instructors, and head nurses. The director has the most influence in this process, however, as he or she is the one to negotiate these goals and objectives with the hospital administrator.

After the organizational goals are established, the director of nursing services and the head nurse may develop a contract for a specific nursing unit. Included in the head nurse's contract may be goals related to areas such as budget and staffing (productivity), quality patient care (quality assurance), staff job satisfaction, and personal growth and development. The head nurse then may negotiate with the various support services for activities which will assist the meeting of these goals. In the same manner, a head nurse may contract with an assistant head nurse or staff nurse to reach a mutual goal.

Contracts are discussed in further detail in Chapter 6.


## SUMMARY

A key element in El Camino's organization is assurance that our patients receive consistently excellent care. The quality of nursing care is a consideration in any nursing structure, but in the traditional nursing organization the assessment of quality usually rests with the director of nursing and the ability to monitor through various methods those under the director's control.

It is the nurse at the bedside who is the foundation of El Camino's nursing service. Perhaps this has been overemphasized. Like any organization, the nursing service is a group of individuals working together toward a common goal. Any organization produces its highest level of service when its members are satisfied and growing. An organization works best toward these goals when it realizes individually and collectively that it is part of a larger world. Yet it cannot discharge its responsibility for care unless it is able to make each individual within the organization aware of the importance of his or her own part within the group. The structure of our nursing organization, then, is based on these premises:

- The individual nurse works best when she or he is responsible, accountable, and free to communicate with any other member of the nursing service.
- Nursing care is centered at the bedside, not in the nursing director's office.
- Care is best achieved in an atmosphere where participation and communication are not only *encouraged* but *required* of each nurse.

# 3

---

# *Staffing:*
# *Stretching Dollars and Talent*

Under decentralized nursing, staffing becomes the responsibility of the head nurse. Each of the 16 nursing units at El Camino Hospital plans for and carries out its own staffing. Other hospital departments assist in the planning and help with support for staffing decisions, but the responsibility for seeing that a unit has adequate staff to render quality nursing care rests with the unit's head nurse.

This staffing program evolved with the inception of decentralization at the hospital. Three factors made it clear that staffing would have to be done at the unit level:

1. *Philosophy.* It is a basic premise of decentralization that the head nurse assumes as much responsibility as possible for the operation of his or her unit.
2. *Economy.* Decentralization's emphasis on unit budget preparation necessitates that staffing and decisions for allocation of personnel be carried out at the unit level.
3. *Communication.* Staffing at the unit level offers an opportunity to improve communication and work relationships between the head nurse and staff nurses on a unit. This is as it should be, for the head nurse is the most qualified to work with the nurses who give the care for which she or he is responsible.

## A STAFFING TASK FORCE LOOKS AT THE PROBLEM

With these factors in mind, a special task force was formed early in the development of decentralization to consider unit-staffing guidelines. The committee consisted of head nurses, budget and recruitment coordinators, a representative of staff development, and the director of nursing services. The task force developed a series of philosophical statements from which staffing goals and policies evolved.


## Philosophy of Staffing

*We believe the staffing needs of El Camino Hospital can best be met by identifying individual patient needs as reflected in the patient dependency system.*

Each head nurse with the support and help from the budget and staffing coordinator and a management engineer develops a patient-dependency system based on that unit's patient care needs over 24 hours. This enables nursing units to base staffing needs on actual patient requirements.

The head nurse implements and continually evaluates the system and is responsible for monitoring the system and the patient-care plans.

*We believe the highest quality care is best provided by people with appropriate skills assigned and committed to a clinical area.*

The head nurse establishes the average staffing requirement for each shift based on historical data (core staffing), and, with assistant head nurses, coordinates the schedules for the unit on a 24-hour basis.

Head nurses in like areas (Critical Care, Maternal-Child-Health, Medical-Surgical-Orthopedic) coordinate vacations, leaves-of-absence, and other planned staffing changes with one another on a regular basis.

The head nurse supplements core staffing from the float pool established for a complex. Complex float pools increase the availability of skilled people for clinical areas and allow for continuity of patient care.

The assignment of float nurses to a specific unit and a specific complex supports their professional growth through the educational opportunities available in the clinical areas. It also increases their commitment to unit standards and improves communication between the float nurses and the unit. The head nurse of the float nurse's assigned unit is responsible for his or her job performance review and evaluation.

*We believe that the head nurse is accountable for decisions regarding selection and utilization of clinical unit personnel.*

The necessary resources and support services are provided to assist the head nurse in personnel decisions.

The Coordinator for nurse recruitment and personnel relations provides recruitment services and initial screening of applicants.

The head nurse communicates anticipated personnel changes to the budget and staffing coordinator. Positions available in nursing service are visually displayed on the staffing board in the staffing office, and all open positions are announced regularly in the *Green Sheet*. Written applications are accepted prior to the announced deadline date. The selection of an individual to fill any clinical unit position is based on the needs of the patients, the needs of the unit, and the qualifications of the applicants.

The nursing administration, the coordinator for nurse recruitment and personnel relations, and the personnel department provide employee-relations resources to head nurses.

The head nurse utilizes all available resources for unit management. These include management support coordinators, management engineering, labor analysis sheets, time cards, admission and discharge data, patient dependency summaries, and the daily staffing reports.

### Determining Numbers

The staffing task force looked first at how a head nurse determines the required number of staff. Of course, the most obvious criterion is that the number of nurses on a given nursing unit be adequate to render high-quality cost-effective patient care.

It is easy to state this premise but difficult to arrive at the precise nurses-to-patient ratio that will ensure its practice. Not all units care for the same types of patients and patient-care requirements on some units are higher than on others. However, the number of patients on any unit and amount of care required tends to vary from day to day.

Before decentralization, these questions were answered from a central nursing office, usually by nursing supervisors who attempted to keep an eye on several different units. Based on their estimates, nurses were assigned from the nursing office.

In effecting our change, we studied past patient-census figures, not only throughout the hospital, but also on individual units. Medical records revealed previous medical-to-surgical case ratios that might be indicative of future admissions. The average length of stay in recent years was determined, and from a random sampling we evaluated the types of patients who had been cared for. Patient figures for different times of the year and different days of the week were studied and analyzed. We looked at discharges and admissions as they related to seasons, months of the year, and days of the week. The number and kinds of Emergency Room cases were studied.

From these analyses emerged definite cyclical patterns. In some units, certain weekdays were likely to show higher figures than others. Seasonal variations could be detected: Fewer patients were admitted to the hospital shortly before Christmas, for example, but the hospital census tended to rise after the first of the year. Admissions continued to increase until about Easter, when it leveled off.

**Exhibit 3-1.   El Camino Hospital District Bi-Weekly Time Schedule**

Station __CCU__

Week of _____

| Name | Class. | Sun | Mon | Tue | Wed | Thu | Fri | Sat | Sun | Mon | Tue | Wed | Thu | Fri | Sat | Total |
|---|---|---|---|---|---|---|---|---|---|---|---|---|---|---|---|---|
| 5/5 | AHN | D | / | / | / | / | D | D | / | D | / | / | / | PTO | D | |
| 5/5 | RN | / | / | D | / | / | / | P | D | D | / | / | / | D | / | |
| 4/5 | RN | / | / | D | D | / | D | D | D | D | / | / | D | / | / | |
| 4/5 | RN | D | D | / | / | D | / | / | D | D | D | / | P | P | D | |
| 3/5 | RN | / | / | D | D | D | / | D | D | D | D | D | D | / | / | |
| 3/5 | RN | / | D | / | D | D | / | D | D | / | / | D | D | D | / | |
| 2/5 | RIV. | D | D | / | D | D | D | / | / | / | / | D | D | D | / | |
| PD | RN | | | | | | | | | | | | | | | |
| 5/5 | Sec. | | | | | | | | | | | | | | | |
| | | | | | | | | | | | | | | | | |
| CORE | | 4 | 4 | 4 | 4 | 4 | 4 | 4 | 4 | 4 | 4 | 4 | 4 | 4 | 4 | |
| ACTUAL | | 4 | 4/1 | 4/1 | 4/1 | 4/1 | 4 | 4 | 4 | 4/1 | 4/1 | 4/1 | 4/1 | 4/1 | | |

PTO = PAID TIME OFF

These, of course, were not the only factors that influenced the hospital census. Something as obscure as the staff cardiac surgeon's decision to go skiing in midweek had its effect on nurse staffing requirements in the operating room and intensive care unit.

Medical conventions, especially those of the medical specialities, affected the number of hospital admissions. Such events as strikes or the possibility of strikes in the community, layoffs because of a downturn in business, and school vacations all were found to be influential.

Demographic data pertaining to the community was considered important in predicting future hospital needs. Age of the population, for example, gave some indication of the number of patients and kinds of illnesses and injuries to expect. Such a seemingly unrelated trend as a rise in the cost of housing might reduce the number of families with children and lower the future pediatric census.

The development of all this information into a coherent pattern eventually provided a set of numerical statistics on which head nurses could base their estimated needs for staff.

Along with consideration of patient census went consideration of cost. Unit staffing must be conducted within the head nurse's specified budget. The combination of these two kinds of data ultimately produced what we call a *core-staffing pattern.*

## Core Staffing

The core staffing reflects the number of staff necessary to care for the number of patients forecast for a given unit. These staff-requirement figures become the unit's master time schedule. Each head nurse or assistant head nurse must use these figures to submit the unit's plans for the coming two weeks. The number of budgeted staff is expressed as full-time equivalent positions. They can divide their personnel into various combinations of full-and part-time positions if they wish. The important thing about the figures is that they provide realistic staffing guidelines.

Exhibit 3-1 is a sample time schedule for El Camino Hospital's Coronary Care Unit (CCU). The clinical unit secretary is scheduled Monday through Friday. Its core-staffing pattern is four full-time staff nurses for each day of the week. The first column of the scheduling sheet normally lists the names of the nurses regularly employed on the unit. It also shows their time commitment. The second column indicates the job category. Because this particular sheet is for an evening shift, it indicates an assistant head nurse, seven registered nurses and a clinical unit secretary. The assistant head nurse and one staff nurse work full time, two nurses work four-fifths time, two work three-fifths time, and one works two-fifths time. Another nurse works per diem. The per-diem status is defined as one that usually does not have a regularly assigned work schedule.

In planning how to use these personnel, the assistant head nurse must take into account each nurse's days off (designated by a "D" on the schedule). Also to be considered are leaves of absence, sickness, and any other factors which may diminish the number of nurses available to work.

By appropriately entering whether or not the individual members of the staff are present on any given day, the head nurse (or in this case, the assistant head nurse) is able to tell whether staff will be available on each of the days of the two-week period. This set of figures can be compared with the core-staffing pattern developed for the unit. A two-week planning period was chosen because it coincides with the hospital's regular pay interval. With all the information properly assembled and written on it, this time schedule is sent to the nursing staffing secretaries.

There are two full-time staffing secretaries; one assigned to work from 6 A.M. to 2:30 P.M., the other from 2 P.M. to 10:30 P.M. Staffing secretaries type time schedules, providing additional copies to head nurses when needed. They post sick calls, excused absence days, and changes in skill status. They are also responsible for completing float schedules after unit requirements have been determined, and for assigning float personnel as they are needed. In general, the staffing secretaries keep a close rein on the number of staff required and the number of staff available, calling additional staff when needed and notifying units when they have sufficient personnel to allow for paid time off or excused absences. Because both secretaries have typing skills, they are available to support most of the head nurses' and assistant head nurses' typing needs.

## PATIENT-DEPENDENCY SYSTEM (ACUITY SYSTEM)

Concurrently with decentralization, a patient-dependency (or acuity) system was established at El Camino Hospital to identify patient-care requirements for each nursing shift. Under such a system the care requirements for each patient are assessed and assigned a numeric acuity. This enables each nursing unit to base its staffing needs on the actual patient load at any given time, thereby ensuring a proper ratio of nurses to patients.

Various dependency-system methodologies are used at El Camino, each designed to meet the appropriate needs of the individual nursing unit.

The acuity scale in the Medical-Surgical-Orthopedic complex ranges from one to four, with patients who are categorized ones needing the least care and patients who are categorized fours needing the most. Surgical unit nurses, for example, assess each patient according to the Surgical Patient Categorization Guidelines (Exhibit 3-2). From the assessment an acuity level of one, two, three, or four is assigned. The number of patients in each category is then matched to the Staff Assignment Guide (see Exhibit 3-3), which indicates the number of staff required to care for those patients. This often is a subjective decision on the part of the nurse caring for the patient. Patient care needs frequently fall into different categories. When this occurs, the nurse must choose the category that best reflects the individual needs of the patient.

Exhibit 3-4 indicates that the night shift on 2-West has acuitized for four patients in category one, which will require .5 staff to care for them. The total number of patients on the unit in all categories is 24, requiring a staff of 5.4 to care for them. On the right-hand side of the form the unit is able to indicate the staff scheduled to work and any known absences. The section "walking or running," which is another way of noting if the unit has too much or too little staff, indicates whether additional staff may be necessary.

The acuity systems for Critial Care, Maternity, Labor and Delivery, and Nursery are somewhat different, but they accomplish the same goal—i.e., an adequate nurse-patient ratio is ensured.

In Critical Care units, an objective point system is used. Points are assigned for various procedures required during any eight-hour shift. Points are matched on a table indicating the staff required for such care. For example, in ICU for other than patients requiring one-to-one care, routine care points for patients on the day shift are 39. This takes into account all the basic nursing care required by ICU patients. Additional points are assigned according to individual patient needs. For example, all ICU patients are on monitors and require emotional support, so each is given five points in those areas. (When acuities are updated, they will likely be included under routine care points.)

The ICU Staffing Summary shown in Exhibit 3-5 indicates that ICU has five patients. We see that Mr. Jones has been given the routine care points (39), is on a monitor (5 points), and requires emotional support (5 points). It is estimated that Mr. Jones will require suctioning at least three times during the next shift, so two points are added for each time. It is also expected that he will be weaned from the respirator, requiring a total of four points, two each time he is taken off and put back on the respirator for the day shift. Mr. Jones has a total of 59 points and the ICU Staff Assignment Guide shows that he requires .74 staff to take care of him. By comparing the total number of patient-care points to the ICU Staff Assignment Guide, we find a total required staff of 3.67. Added to that are the unit secretary and the nurse (or nurses) required for a one-to-one patient. ICU's total staff required for our sample day is 5.67. Also on the Staffing Summary is space to indicate the scheduled staff as well as absences.

A similar system is used in Nursery, Maternity, and Transitional Care. The point assignments are different, but the matching of tasks to personnel is much the same. No matter which of these systems is used, the total of acuities must be matched to the number of patients on the unit.

Predicting patient needs has proved to be a difficult and often frustrating challenge. We are still looking for a better system, one that can predict more accurately the many facets of care that our patients require and the time it takes to render such care. Our system has evolved over the years; we agree that

**Exhibit 3-2.    Surgical Patient Categorization Guidelines**

| | I | II | III | IV |
|---|---|---|---|---|
| **Treatments** | Simple dressing changes and/or reinforcement. Test procedure preparation requiring brief explanation and/or one medication, VS, checking circulation or color once/shift. ROM and/or neuro checks once/shift. | Any 1 tmt. more than once/shift. FC care, I&O, bladder irrigations, sitz bath, compresses, tests preps req. more than one med and/or involved exploration. Enema for evacuation, Harris flush, assist MD with procedures, i.e., bone marrow, sigmoidoscopy, LP, liver biopsy, epidural injection, decubitus care Stage I&II, S&As, application of pelvic or cervical traction. | VS, neuro checks on ROM more than twice/shift. Complicated dressings or wound irrigations, care of tracheotomy, suctioning, cannula care, hyperalimentation dressing changes, chest tubes, CVP arteriogram (1st day). | Extensive dressings requiring frequent changes. Patients on Stryker frames, VS, neuro cks or ROM more than Q2hr. Assisting MD with amniocentesis, D&C on the unit, delivery of a fetus. Frequent treatments such as irrigating post-TUR bleeders, iced lavage. Reverse or strict isolation. Decubitus care Stage III, 1st and 2nd day colostomy irrigation, hypothermia. |
| **Medications** | Simple, routine, or PRN medications once/shift. No IVs. No pre- or post-med needing evaluation. | Two of the following types of medication: diabetic, cardiac, hypo- & hypertensive, diuretic or anticoagulant. PRNs twice/shift. Volutrol meds once/shift. IVs (medicated & non-medicated). Oral chemotherapy pre/post- med needing eval. | More than two of category II medications and PRNs more than twice/shift. Volutrol meds twice/shift. Continuous medicated wound irrigations. | More intensive category III medications. PRNs given Q1H or more often. Hyperalimentation, blood transfusions, platelets, IV, Pitocin. Volutrol meds more than twice/shift. IV chemotherapy. |

| | | | |
|---|---|---|---|
| **Emotional Support** | Patient needing support related simply to being hospitalized. | Patient who has difficulty with English language. Simple discharge planning involving family. Mild adverse reaction to illness—depression, anxiety, insomnia. | Patient whose emotional needs are severe but are being met according to the patient care plan. The patient who speaks no English or is passively confused. Discharge planning involving other agencies and including a patient care plan. | Emotional needs are severe and are not being met by the care plan. Aphasic patients or those who are disoriented and combative. |
| **Teaching** | Pre- & post-op teaching for minor surgeries or procedures | Pre- & post-op teaching for major surgeries or procedures. Simple discharge teaching. | Teaching of care of ostomies, new diabetics, conditions requiring major changes in ADL. Pre-op teaching for total hip, post-op teaching for supra pubic catheters (day 1 only), complex discharge teaching. | Patient unable or unwilling to learn—all teaching must be done with significant others. |
| **Documentation of Patient Status** | Routine charting. Routine updating of care plan. | Charting against 1–2 EO. Initial care planning. Admission interview. Care planning with 1–2 problems. | Charting against 3–4 EO. Care planning with 3–4 problems. | Charting against 4 + EO. Care planning with 4 + problems. |

**Exhibit 3-2.** *(continued)*

| | I | II | III | IV |
|---|---|---|---|---|
| **Eating** | Needs little help. Feeds self. | Needs some help in preparing food for eating. May need encouragement. 1–2-hr. ulcer regime feedings. Monitoring patient's response to new diet. | Needs feeding. Routine tube feedings. | Tube feedings 2 hr. |
| **Grooming** | Takes own shower, tub or sponge bath. | Does own bath but needs assistance with back and feet. Needs setting up with oral hygiene, hair combing, etc. | Needs complete bed bath but able to move self with minimal assistance. | Patient unable to assist with any part of bath. |
| **Excretion** | BRP without assistance | Needs assistance in getting up to bathroom or using urinal. (For patients with Foleys, refer to treatment category). Assist with colostomy/ileostomy bag changing. 24-hr. urine collection. | In bed needing bedpan or urinal placed and removed. May be able to turn or lift self. Assist with bag changing and irrigation for patients with ostomies. Commode or occas. incont. | Completely dependent. Unable to ask for bedpan or urinal. (Incontinent). |

| | | | | |
|---|---|---|---|---|
| **Physical Comfort** | Able to adjust position or bed by self. | Needs assistance with adjustment of position of bed (tubes, IVs pelvic traction, upper extremity casts). Transport to PT, etc. once/shift. Amb. without assist. | Cannot turn without help, getting drink, adjust position of extremities, etc. (lower extremity casts and those who need help in getting into a chair or commode or with crutch walking.) Transport to PT, etc. twice/shift. | Completely dependent. Needs complete assistance in changing position. Needs more than 2 people to transfer to chair or commode. Hoyer lift needed. Log rolling. |
| **General Health** | General health is good. In for diagnostic procedure, simple treatment. Pre-op minor surgery, i.e., D&C, biopsy, minor fractures, etc. | Pre-op major surgeries, post myelograms, more than one illness. Post MI who is convalescing. Post-op minor surgeries (day of surgery). Pre-op minor surgeries who are AM admits. | Arteriograms with frequent VS. Post-op major surgeries (day of surgery). Post-cardiac cath., liver biopsies, kidney biopsies. Brittle diabetics, day 1&2 post CVA. Pre-op cataracts. | Critically ill. Terminal illness with impending death. |

*Advance to next category for isolation.

**Exhibit 3-3.    Staff Assignment Guide (MSO)**

STAFF REQUIRED PER SHIFT

| NO. OF PTS. | DAYS | | | | EVENINGS | | | | NIGHTS | | | |
|---|---|---|---|---|---|---|---|---|---|---|---|---|
| | 1 | 2 | 3 | 4 | 1 | 2 | 3 | 4 | 1 | 2 | 3 | 4 |
| 1 | .2 | .3 | .3 | .5 | .1 | .2 | .3 | .4 | .1 | .1 | .2 | .2 |
| 2 | .3 | .5 | .7 | 1.0 | .3 | .4 | .6 | .8 | .2 | .2 | .3 | .5 |
| 3 | .5 | .8 | 1.0 | 1.5 | .4 | .6 | .8 | 1.2 | .2 | .3 | .5 | .7 |
| 4 | .7 | 1.0 | 1.4 | 2.0 | .5 | .8 | 1.1 | 1.7 | .3 | .5 | .6 | .9 |
| 5 | .8 | 1.3 | 1.7 | 2.5 | .7 | 1.0 | 1.4 | 2.1 | .4 | .6 | .8 | 1.2 |
| 6 | 1.0 | 1.5 | 2.1 | 3.0 | .8 | 1.2 | 1.7 | 2.5 | .5 | .7 | .9 | 1.4 |
| 7 | 1.2 | 1.8 | 2.4 | 3.6 | .9 | 1.5 | 2.0 | 2.9 | .5 | .8 | 1.1 | 1.6 |
| 8 | 1.3 | 2.0 | 2.7 | 4.1 | 1.1 | 1.7 | 2.2 | 3.4 | .6 | .9 | 1.2 | 1.8 |
| 9 | 1.5 | 2.3 | 3.1 | 4.6 | 1.2 | 1.9 | 2.5 | 3.7 | .7 | 1.0 | 1.4 | 2.1 |
| 10 | 1.6 | 2.5 | 3.4 | 5.1 | 1.3 | 2.1 | 2.8 | 4.2 | .8 | 1.2 | 1.6 | 2.3 |
| 11 | 1.8 | 2.8 | 3.8 | 5.6 | 1.5 | 2.3 | 3.1 | 4.6 | .8 | 1.3 | 1.7 | 2.5 |
| 12 | 2.0 | 3.0 | 4.1 | 6.1 | 1.6 | 2.5 | 3.4 | 5.0 | .9 | 1.4 | 1.9 | 2.8 |
| 13 | 2.1 | 3.3 | 4.5 | 6.6 | 1.8 | 2.7 | 3.6 | 5.4 | 1.0 | 1.5 | 2.0 | 3.0 |
| 14 | 2.3 | 3.6 | 4.8 | 7.1 | 1.9 | 2.9 | 3.9 | 5.8 | 1.1 | 1.6 | 2.2 | 3.2 |
| 15 | 2.5 | 3.8 | 5.1 | 7.6 | 2.0 | 3.1 | 4.2 | 6.2 | 1.1 | 1.7 | 2.3 | 3.5 |
| 16 | 2.6 | 4.1 | 5.5 | 8.1 | 2.2 | 3.3 | 4.5 | 6.6 | 1.2 | 1.8 | 2.5 | 3.7 |
| 17 | 2.8 | 4.3 | 5.8 | 8.6 | 2.3 | 3.5 | 4.8 | 7.1 | 1.3 | 2.0 | 2.6 | 3.9 |
| 18 | 3.0 | 4.6 | 6.2 | 9.1 | 2.4 | 3.7 | 5.0 | 7.5 | 1.4 | 2.1 | 2.8 | 4.2 |
| 19 | 3.1 | 4.8 | 6.5 | 9.6 | 2.6 | 3.9 | 5.3 | 7.9 | 1.4 | 2.2 | 3.0 | 4.4 |
| 20 | 3.3 | 5.1 | 6.9 | 10.2 | 2.7 | 4.2 | 5.6 | 8.3 | 1.5 | 2.3 | 3.1 | 4.6 |
| 21 | 3.5 | 5.3 | 7.2 | 10.7 | 2.8 | 4.4 | 5.9 | 8.7 | 1.6 | 2.4 | 3.3 | 4.8 |
| 22 | 3.6 | 5.6 | 7.5 | 11.2 | 3.0 | 4.6 | 6.2 | 9.1 | 1.7 | 2.5 | 3.4 | 5.1 |
| 23 | 3.8 | 5.8 | 7.9 | 11.7 | 3.1 | 4.8 | 6.4 | 9.5 | 1.7 | 2.7 | 3.6 | 5.3 |
| 24 | 4.0 | 6.1 | 8.2 | 12.2 | 3.2 | 5.0 | 6.7 | 10.0 | 1.8 | 2.8 | 3.7 | 5.5 |
| 25 | 4.1 | 6.3 | 8.6 | 12.7 | 3.4 | 5.2 | 7.0 | 10.4 | 1.9 | 2.9 | 3.9 | 5.8 |

**Exhibit 3-4. Nursing Unit Staffing Summary**

RETURN TO STAFFING OFFICE
BY: 5:00 AM

NURSING UNIT: _2 WEST_      DATE: _____

PREPARED BY: _____

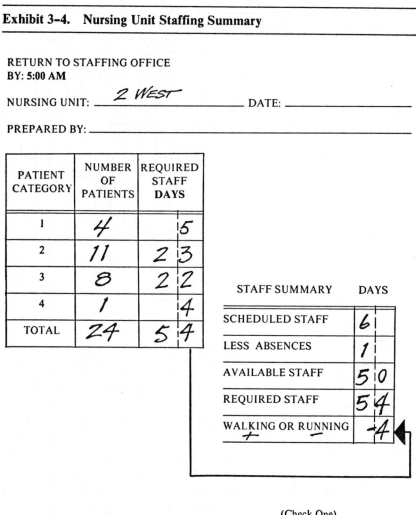

| PATIENT CATEGORY | NUMBER OF PATIENTS | REQUIRED STAFF DAYS |
|---|---|---|
| 1 | 4 | 5 |
| 2 | 11 | 23 |
| 3 | 8 | 22 |
| 4 | 1 | 4 |
| TOTAL | 24 | 54 |

| STAFF SUMMARY | DAYS |
|---|---|
| SCHEDULED STAFF | 6 |
| LESS ABSENCES | 1 |
| AVAILABLE STAFF | 50 |
| REQUIRED STAFF | 54 |
| WALKING OR RUNNING | -4 |

| NAMES OF ABSENTEES | ILL. | (Check One) HOL. | VAC. | EA. |
|---|---|---|---|---|
| SUE JONES | ✓ | | | |
| | | | | |
| | | | | |
| | | | | |

COMMENTS: _O.K._

## Exhibit 3-5.  ICU Staffing Summary

DATE: _____    PREPARED FOR:  DAY ☐   EVENING ☐   NIGHT ☐

PREPARED BY:

| ACTIVITIES | POINTS | Smith 1 | Jones 2 | Brown 3 | Long 4 | 5 | Green 6 | 7 | 8 | 9 | 10 | 11 | 12 | 13 | 14 | 15 | 16 |
|---|---|---|---|---|---|---|---|---|---|---|---|---|---|---|---|---|---|
| Monitor | 5 | 5 | 5 | 5 | 5 | | 5 | | | | | | | | | | |
| Suctioning (ea.) | 2 | | 6 | 16 | | | | | | | | | | | | | |
| Weaning (ea.) | 2 | | 4 | | | | | | | | | | | | | | |
| Blood gas; cardiac output | 4 | 4 | | 4 | | | | | | | | | | | | | |
| Tube feeding (ea.) | 2 | | | | | | | | | | | | | | | | |
| Procedure off unit | 10 | | | | | | | | | | | | | | | | |
| Bedscale weight | 6 | | | | | | | | | | | | | | | | |
| Incontinence (ea.) | 4 | | | | | | | | | | | | | | | | |
| Assist with procedure | 10 | | | | | | | | | | | | | | | | |
| Freq. V/S (hemodynamic) | 5/10 | 5 | | | | | | | | | | | | | | | |
| Freq. V/S (s̄ art. line) | 20 | | | | | | | | | | | | | | | | |
| Admit patient | 10 | | | | | | | | | | | | | | | | |
| Transfer patient | 10 | | | | 10 | | | | | | | | | | | | |
| Emotional support | 5 | 5 | 5 | 5 | 5 | | 5 | | | | | | | | | | |
| Patient teaching | 5 | | | | | | | | | | | | | | | | |
| | | | | | | | | | | | | | | | | | |
| | | | | | | | | | | | | | | | | | |
| | | | | | | | | | | | | | | | | | |
| Routine care points* | | 39 | 39 | 39 | 39 | | 39 | | | | | | | | | | |
| | | | | | | | | | | | | | | | | | |
| | | | | | | | | | | | | | | | | | |

* 7-3  3-11
  39    31
  11-7
  31

| | | Smith 1 | Jones 2 | Brown 3 | Long 4 | 5 | Green 6 | 7 | 8 | 9 | 10 | 11 | 12 | 13 | 14 | 15 | 16 |
|---|---|---|---|---|---|---|---|---|---|---|---|---|---|---|---|---|---|
| TOTAL POINTS | | 58 | 59 | 69 | 59 | | 49 | | | | | | | | | | |
| REQUIRED STAFF | | .72 | .74 | .86 | .74 | | .61 | | | | | | | | | | |

| | | |
|---|---|---|
| TOTAL REQUIRED STAFF | 3 | 67 |
| 1:1 PATIENTS | 1 | 00 |
| CLERK | 1 | 00 |
| CONST. ATTEND. RELIEF (.2) | | |
| PRE-OP TEACH (.1) | | |
| TOTAL STAFF REQUIRED | 5 | 67 |

| STAFF SUMMARY | STAFF | |
|---|---|---|
| Scheduled Staff | 7 | 00 |
| Sick Calls/Absences | 1 | 00 |
| Available Staff | 6 | 00 |
| Less Required | 5 | 67 |
| Over, or Under | | 67 |
| Floats In, Out EAs | 1 to TOU | |
| FINAL STAFF: | 5 | 00 |

### 1:1 PATIENT CATEGORIES

- Post-op open heart
- Complete isolation
- Peritoneal dialysis
- Confused, restless, needing constant attention

Form No. 931   Revised 10/78, ICU Staff, JF

## Exhibit 3-6.  Intensive Care Units Staff Assignment Guide

| Patient Points | Staff | Patient Points | Staff | Patient Points | Staff |
|---|---|---|---|---|---|
| 20 | .25 | 51 | .64 | 81 | 1.01 |
| 21 | .26 | 52 | .65 | 82 | 1.02 |
| 22 | .27 | 53 | .66 | 83 | 1.04 |
| 23 | .29 | 54 | .67 | 84 | 1.05 |
| 24 | .30 | 55 | .69 | 85 | 1.06 |
| 25 | .31 | 56 | .70 | 86 | 1.07 |
| 26 | .32 | 57 | .71 | 87 | 1.09 |
| 27 | .34 | 58 | .72 | 88 | 1.10 |
| 28 | .35 | 59 | .74 | 89 | 1.11 |
| 29 | .36 | 60 | .75 | 90 | 1.12 |
| 30 | .37 | 61 | .76 | 91 | 1.14 |
| 31 | .39 | 62 | .77 | 92 | 1.15 |
| 32 | .40 | 63 | .79 | 93 | 1.16 |
| 33 | .41 | 64 | .80 | 94 | 1.17 |
| 34 | .42 | 65 | .81 | 95 | 1.19 |
| 35 | .44 | 66 | .82 | 96 | 1.20 |
| 36 | .45 | 67 | .84 | 97 | 1.21 |
| 37 | .46 | 68 | .85 | 98 | 1.22 |
| 38 | .47 | 69 | .86 | 99 | 1.24 |
| 39 | .49 | 70 | .87 | 100 | 1.25 |
| 40 | .50 | 71 | .89 | 101 | 1.26 |
| 41 | .51 | 72 | .90 | 102 | 1.27 |
| 42 | .52 | 73 | .91 | 103 | 1.29 |
| 43 | .54 | 74 | .92 | 104 | 1.30 |
| 44 | .55 | 75 | .94 | 105 | 1.31 |
| 45 | .56 | 76 | .95 | 106 | 1.32 |
| 46 | .57 | 77 | .96 | 107 | 1.34 |
| 47 | .59 | 78 | .97 | 108 | 1.35 |
| 48 | .60 | 79 | .99 | 109 | 1.36 |
| 49 | .61 | 80 | 1.00 | 110 | 1.37 |
| 50 | .62 | | | | |

---

**Exhibit 3-7.    Admitting/Staffing Sheet**

---

DATE _____    SHIFT _____

| UNIT | CENSUS | PLUS (+) | MINUS (-) | COMMENTS |
|------|--------|----------|-----------|----------|
| MATERNITY | | | | |
| 2 NORTH | | | | |
| PEDIATRICS | | | | |
| 2 WEST | | | | |
| 2 EAST | | | | |
| 3 WEST | | | | |
| 5 WEST | | | | |
| 5 EAST | | | | |
| 6 WEST | | | | |
| 6 EAST | | | | |

it's far from perfect and needs to be constantly updated, but it has provided us the tools necessary to improve and monitor the utilization of nursing personnel.

Acuity reports are sent to the nursing staffing office at noon, eight P.M., and five A.M. There the staffing secretary coordinates the staffing of the Medical-Surgical-Orthopedic units and Maternal-Child-Health units for the oncoming shift. The Critical-Care complex coordinates its own staffing, but it confers with the staffing secretaries in situations of over- or understaffing. In this way a nurse has the option of floating to another complex where additional personnel are needed—provided, of course, that the available floater has the necessary skills. At this time the staffing secretary completes the Admitting/Staffing Sheet (Exhibit 3-7) and forwards it to the admitting department.

This form reflects the census level on each of the MSO and MCH units. It includes information about each unit's staffing, indicating how much they may be over or under their staffing requirements for that shift.

This information can be a useful tool in deciding where unscheduled emergency admissions should be assigned. The workload can be more evenly distributed by admitting patients to areas better staffed to care for them.

## Staffing Board

In the staffing office a large board reflects the assignment location of every nurse in the hospital. A slip containing each nurse's name and skill level is posted beneath the name of her assigned unit.

The staffing board also includes the number of budgeted positions for each unit along with the names of the unit's head nurse and assistant head nurses. Units are grouped according to complex: Maternal-Child-Health, Medical-Surgical-Orthopedic, and Critical Care. Shifts are denoted and nurses on leaves of absence or sick leave have appropriate tags added to their names. By color coding the different tags, it also is possible to denote those nurses certified in cardiopulmonary resuscitation, chemotherapy, and other specialties.

In short, a look at the board reveals the entire staffing situation, not only for individual units, but also for the hospital as a whole. This allows the staffing office to note where gaps exist in staffing and makes it possible for head nurses to determine available staff, should they need help. The board also makes easily visible the number of nurses in the float pool, how and where they may be shifted, and how nursing staffing in general may relate to the hospital census.

Head nurses and their assistants are encouraged to examine the board at least once a week so they can keep abreast of the situation in the hospital as it develops and relates to their unit.

## Float Personnel

The philosophy of decentralization maximizes unit staffing and minimizes a centralized float pool. Therefore there are few float personnel at El Camino. However, to provide for effective communication and evaluation with and among this comparatively small group of float personnel, it was necessary to establish some permanent means of integrating them into the nursing service. It became apparent that they, too, needed a unit with which to identify for the purposes of problem solving, evaluation, and communication. This was solved by setting up float pools and assigning each float person to a specific head nurse and unit. There is a Critical Care float pool and a combined Medical-Surgical-Orthopedic and Maternal-Child-Health float pool. A separate MCH float pool would be impractical, as few floats are used in these units. The majority of MSO/MCH floats are cross-trained to allow greater flexibility.

A separate float budget assumes the cost of float orientation, preceptor time, and paid time off. When float personnel are used, they are sent to areas where there has been an unexpected sick call that the unit is unable to fill or where unusually high acuities have been recorded.

## COMPLEX CAPTAINS

As decentralization progressed, a system involving "complex captains" was developed. The head nurses within a complex serve in this capacity on a rotational basis, assuming specific administrative management and budget/staffing responsibilities on the complex level.

The administrative responsibilities of complex captains are as follows:

To communicate their identity and length of rotation as captain to the staffing office.
To act as complex resource person for the director of nursing services, department heads, coordinators, staff development people, etc.
To manage the weekly complex meetings, either chairing them personally or delegating the chairmanship; to plan and coordinate the agenda and keep the minutes.
To follow up any action plans and communications flow generated in the complex meetings.
(In Maternal-Child-Health complex only) To serve as a member of the Executive Advisory Committee.

The budget and staffing functions and responsibilities of complex captains are as follows:

To review regularly with the budget and staffing coordinator the float positions on the staffing board.
To advertise open float positions in the Nursing Newsletter.
To review applications and hire for the position.
To coordinate the orientation of new float nurses, assigning them to specific head/assistant-head nurses within the complex for coaching and development, counseling, performance appraisal, and, when necessary, termination.
To communicate and meet with the staffing secretaries to keep abreast of current staffing situations and complex float utilization.
To finalize float time schedules and float paid time off (PTO) requests.
To make final decisions on the complex's staffing needs and float assignments in times of crisis and/or conflict situations.
In Critical Care the current complex captain's unit is responsible for the coordination of all staffing. Even on shifts when the actual captain is off duty, the assistant head nurse in charge reviews each unit's acuities and staffing and coordinates them. This individual is also responsible for reporting to the staffing secretary the status of all CC units and for securing any additional personnel who may be needed in order to maintain quality patient care.
Complex captains should not be viewed as substitutes for staffing supervisors. Their work is advisory, not supervisory. The task of selecting the nurses needed to staff a unit remains that of the head nurse.
If the staffing secretary has any questions or problems regarding scheduling, he or she will contact the complex captain for assistance in problem identification and solution, which may or may not involve other head nurses.

## RECRUITMENT AND EMPLOYMENT

Recruitment remains a centrally coordinated function. All open positions are advertised in the hospital's weekly Green Sheet. If positions are not filled through this medium, they are advertised externally, usually in the local newspaper or through nursing journals.

### Hiring From Within

Nursing staff are hired onto straight shifts, usually evenings or nights, as opposed to rotating shifts. To ensure opportunity to all nursing staff who desire eventual permanent placement on the day shift, a hiring protocol has been established:

- All nursing service openings are first advertised in The Green Sheet.
- Interested staff members apply in writing to the specified head nurse.
- A direct hire to the day shift may occur *only in the event that no qualified response has been received from within* after a reasonable period of in-house advertising (two weeks).
- The final selection is made by the head nurse, who will consider the needs of the patients, the needs of the unit, and the qualifications of the applicants. All input should be directed to the head nurse.
- Seniority will be the deciding factor in the case of the two candidates with similar or equal qualifications.

### Hiring New Personnel

When outside applicants appear at the hospital, they are first interviewed by the coordinator for nurse recruitment and personnel relations, who screens them and arranges interviews with the appropriate head nurse. She works closely with head nurses and the budget and staffing coordinator. The recruitment coordinator is in charge of maintaining and posting the open positions and works closely with the head nurses as well as with the budget and staffing coordinator. The recruitment coordinator helps interpret work agreements and assists the hospital administration in matters of salary and personnel relations among nurses. When necessary, this individual may also coach head nurses in interviewing techniques. The recruitment coordinator represents the general nursing service at such functions as fair jobs, recruitment trips, career days, and open houses. However, the assessment, planning, and implementing of various recruitment functions is coordinated with representatives from various levels in nursing.

After screening by the recruitment coordinator, qualified applicants are referred to appropriate head nurses for a unit interview. In keeping with the decentralization concept, assistant head nurses are assuming an active role in the selection of personnel for their own shifts. Thus most head nurses include

---

**Exhibit 3-8.   El Camino Hospital Nursing Service**
*Work Agreement*

---

I accept employment at El Camino Hospital with the following understanding. That I:

1.    Must have Health Service clearance prior to hire.
2.    Am being hired to work as a Staff Nurse_____Step_____at_____(salary) starting_____(orientation date). My employee time category will be_____ .
3.    Am being assigned to_____(unit) on_____(shift) and commit myself to work on this unit and shift for a minimum of_____months before requesting a transfer or status change.
4.    Will float from my assigned area as required.
5.    Am being employed on a trial basis for ninety days and that during this period a preceptor will be designated to oversee my orientation and will discuss my progress with me.
6.    Will abide by the Job Description for my position, the rules of conduct as stated in the Employees Handbook and the Nursing Department dress code.
7.    Understand that because of fluctuating patient census, the hospital cannot guarantee that I will work the full number of hours assigned in my category and that there may be times when it will be necessary for me to reschedule holidays or vacations or take time off without pay.
8.    Can obtain information regarding retirement and employee benefits from the Personnel Department.
9.    (Optional) We mutually agree to the following: _____
      _____
      _____
      _____
      _____
      _____

Signature of applicant _____
Date _____
Signature of Head-Nurse _____
Date _____

Original to Personnel
Copy to Employee
PA/hds   10/77

the specific assistant head nurse in the unit interview or set up an additional meeting for the candidate and the assistant. Rarely would a head nurse hire a registered nurse to evening or night shift without first reaching a consensus with the assistant.

## Orientation

Orientation for new nursing personnel is carried out on a hospital-wide basis. Orientation sessions begin twice each month. During the three-week orientation period the new staff nurse codes time to new training and is not counted as part of the staffing requirement for patient care.

## The Individual Work Agreement

Once a prospect has been accepted for a position, the head nurse and her new staff member sit down and negotiate an individual work agreement (Exihibit 3-8). This document does not replace any existing collective bargaining agreement, but it is a formal statement of the agreement reached between the head nurse and the new staff nurse. The agreement may include such items as a work schedule that varies from that of the regular shift, a contract for the length of time the new nurse agrees to work the night or evening shift, certain days off, or methods of accomplishing special education. Other items in the work agreement include necessary health clearance before working, willingness to float as required, a probationary period, and the understanding that full hours may not be worked if the hospital census declines.

Most important, the agreement contains a specific time commitment. This is a pledge that the new staff person will remain on the unit for a designated period. Most head nurses now seek at least a year's commitment from their new hires. While this commitment is more moral than legal, its clear statement of expectations from both parties has helped retention on most units.

## Special Problem Solving

In a decentralized setting, recruitment and retention of nurses becomes a concern and responsibility of all nurse leaders.

At one time, for example, the recurrence of open positions on the Critical Care night shift was identified as a problem. A Critical Care recruitment task force was formed to problem solve the situation. Included on this committee were the director of nursing services, the director of education and training, and the coordinator of nurse recruitment; also critical care instructors, head nurses, and one staff nurse; plus the assistant personnel manager, a public-relations representative, and nursing coordinators from both the evening and night shifts. By using a collective problem-solving technique, this group brainstormed the situation. The generated ideas were categorized into three parts:

- Marketing plans
- Total organization effort
- Working conditions

The group had many ideas about marketing. One that paid off was to increase the opportunity of critical-care inservice and experiences available to our Medical-Surgical-Orthopedic nurses, thereby recruiting from within. Larger advertisements in nursing journals were helpful, as were personal recruitment letters sent by El Camino Hospital nurses to registered nurse friends and colleagues elsewhere. Of course some far-out ideas were mentioned—e.g., sending the coordinator for recruitment to Chicago during a blizzard with pictures of sunny California; or renting the Goodyear Blimp to float the message, "Work at El Camino Hospital!"

Ideas about total organization and working conditions proved just as worthwhile and, at times, just as fun and far-out. Most significant, however, was the idea for a beginning-level critical-care course to be given at El Camino Hospital by our critical-care instructors. To date there have been two series of classes with very satisfactory results. In return for instruction in critical-care skills and the offer of an internship to reinforce their learning, nurses agree to work either the 3–11 or 11–7 shift in Critical Care. This has helped significantly in filling those once-chronic openings.


## TRACKING SYSTEMS

Staff utilization reviews are made with comparative ease at El Camino Hospital. At the end of each pay period the hospital's management-engineering department compares nursing time cards with all unit acuity sheets generated during that two-week period. This means that actual time worked is compared with actual time required. By dividing the number of hours required to care for the patients on a unit by the total number of hours actually worked, a true picture of unit productivity and cost effectiveness can be obtained. This process is specific to the patient-care productivity cost center discussed in Chapter 4.

Each unit has four cost centers to which information is coded: patient care, administrative time, education, and new training. For example, time coded to the administrative cost center includes time that the head nurse or other unit personnel spend on administrative tasks not a part of patient care. Administrative time may include such jobs as preparing and giving employee performance reviews, doing committee work, counseling unit personnel, researching unit problems, preparing time schedules, carrying out unit planning, holding unit conferences, and performing management functions required to keep the unit in operation.

By using cost centers it is possible to identify for purposes of analysis and problem solving how much time is being spent on specific functions within the nursing unit. Cost-center information is important in budgeting, for it tells the nursing service exactly how accurate forecasting and planning have been. And, of course, it helps forecast and plan the coming year.

### The Forecasting Committee

El Camino Hospital established a forecasting committee, whose prime responsibility is to forecast hospital census three weeks ahead of time. The committee includes the admitting-department head (who is a nurse), three hospital administrators, the director of nursing, the nurse scheduler from the operating room, a representative of management engineering, a staffing coordinator, and one head nurse. The admitting department provides the committee with information on how many scheduled admissions the hospital can expect during the three-week period. The operating room nurse tracks surgical activity and scheduled surgeries that will go to the Intensive Care Unit.

The hospital's surgery schedule is a crucial document. If the schedule shows an unusually large number of planned admissions for pediatric surgery, for example, the pediatric unit is notified that it must prepare for additional patients. If the surgical load is likely to fall elsewhere, those units are informed.

Direct admissions scheduled in advance by staff physicians are related by the committee to the number of beds likely to be available. By meeting each Tuesday and Friday, the committee gains some idea of the prospects for unscheduled admissions.

The committee must also consider vacations, such variables as medical conventions, and the seasonal history regarding the likely number of admissions. During periods of extremely high census, the forecasting committee communicates the resulting bed shortage to the medical staff and other hospital employees, and requests that physicians discharge those patients who are able to go home. When the situation returns to normal and the bed situation eases, the forecasting committee informs physicians accordingly.

On Fridays, the forecasting committee tries to make an in-depth prediction of activity for the following two weeks. If it appears that scheduled staff will be insufficient to meet patient needs, then additional staff can be called in to work.

El Camino Hospital is part of a communications network set up and operated by county government. Originally designed as a means of monitoring admissions to county hospitals at the time of disasters, the network now also works to assist hospitals in handling emergency admissions and, when necessary, can monitor the number of emergency admissions. When El Camino Hospital is near capacity, hospital personnel can contact county communications personnel who, by radio or telephone, will divert ambulances to other nearby hospitals.

The control of unscheduled admissions is important because El Camino is a district hospital whose first priority is the taxpayers who contribute to its support. Control also makes possible a very low rate of cancellation of scheduled admissions. If admissions must be cancelled, it is far easier to predict with the forecasting system. However, El Camino Hospital makes every effort to avoid such cancellations, and its record to date in not disrupting the schedules of physicians and patients is good.

All information gathered by the Friday forecasting meeting and other means is displayed on a forecasting board kept in the staffing office. Head nurses are encouraged to examine it when they check the staffing board. It shows at a glance the hospital's predicted census for the next three weeks and it includes information about the types of patients expected.

## SUMMARY

It must be emphasized that none of the steps described in this planning process emerged overnight. Rather, they were achieved through a process of evolution, sometimes through trial and error, and always with consultation and participation by many members of the hospital nursing staff. Participation by many in the process of planning for a workable staffing system has been essential to its success. Indeed, creative scheduling by the head nurse is possible because of the way in which the system has been organized. The fact that head nurses are responsible for staffing their own units makes it infinitely easier for them to see what they need to make their units operate effectively and efficiently. Creative scheduling includes the possibility of arranging nurses' hours outside the rigid three-shift schedule used by so many hospitals. Many El Camino nurses now report for work at different hours. In addition, the use of flexible work weeks has proven staffing value. Some head nurses now allow for a ten-hour, four-day work week; in emergency staffing situations there have, on occasion, been twelve-hour days.

Even as this system evolves, it faces change. Just as the requirements for staff cannot be rigid, so must problem solving be flexible and constantly under review. The fact that El Camino believes in constant monitoring of its system is essential to its success.

A key philosophical foundation of decentralization is that it must be subject to change. This is no less true in staffing than in other parts of the decentralization structure. By agreeing that change is constant and necessary and that participation is required at all levels of the staffing planning process, we have constructed the outlines of a system that will work in the future as well as it does in the present.

Our system centers around the head nurses. It involves their planning; thus it also involves the support of those members of the nursing staff who can provide essential information. But the decisions about how to use the information remain with the head nurse. And that, as much as anything, is at the heart of the decentralized nursing structure.

# 4

*Budgeting:*
*Holding the Purse Strings*

Concern about the spiraling cost of health care is a recurrent theme in discussions, debates, and analyses of national economic trends. Politicians, their constituents, the consumers of health care, and—most notably—the governmental and private agencies responsible for paying the bills for health care all have observed with consternation a quadrupling of costs in the last few years. It is believed that these costs have contributed significantly to a skyrocketing national inflation. This one belief has stimulated the passage of much federal and state legislation, directing the providers of health care to cut costs, improve utilization, increase productivity, reduce unnecessary services, plan appropriately, coordinate delivery, and assure quality. These were some of Mary Smithwick's findings in her recent master's theses.

## THE BUDGET PROCESS

At El Camino Hospital, this same belief has stimulated development of comprehensive and sophisticated budgeting methods. Nurses had been involved for several years on a rather superficial level in budget preparation when it became evident that the only real way to control costs yet ensure adequate and appropriate human and material resources was to decentralize the budgeting process.

By definition, the budgeting process is a tool for planning, monitoring, and controlling cost. It enables the director of nursing to demonstrate the cost of the nursing care required in each hospital unit. A nursing unit's budgeting process should accomplish the following:

- Plan for required patient hours.
- Plan for paid time off, vacation, holidays, etc.
- Take into account weekends off.

**Exhibit 4-1.  Planning/Budgeting Process**

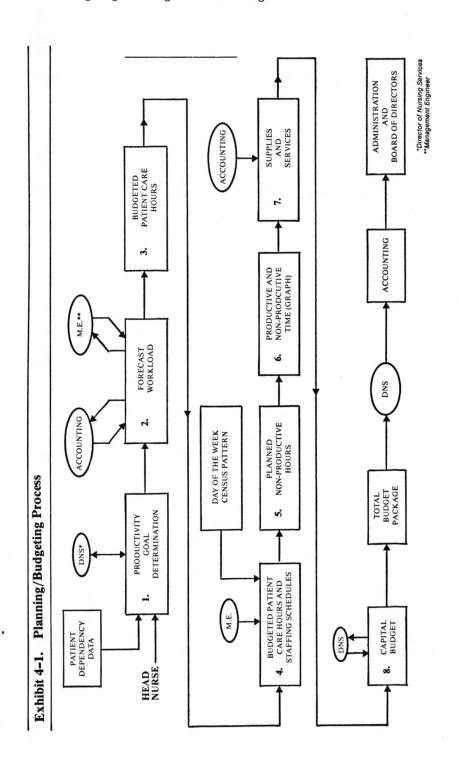

*Director of Nursing Services
**Management Engineer

- Plan for nondirect patient-care activities.
- Correlate budgeted positions to actual day-of-the-week staffing patterns by shift.
- Include measures of performance, both of finances and productivity. (In this case productivity equals the ratio of the required patient-care hours based on the patient census and acuity to the actual hours worked.)

A flow diagram depicting the steps in our budget-planning process is shown in Exhibit 4-1. Nursing service is labor intensive, and this is reflected in the fact that the first six budget-planning steps pertain to that area:

1. *Productivity goal determination:* Here the director of nursing services and the head nurse determine the unit's productivity goal for the coming fiscal year.
2. *Forecast workload:* The number of patient days expected on each nursing unit for the coming fiscal year are forecasted.
3. *Budgeted patient care hours:* The number of hours expected to be used in patient care for the patient days are forecasted.
4. *Budgeted patient care hours and staffing schedules:* Here the budgeted patient care hours are reflected in recommended staffing schedules by shift and by day of the week.
5. *Planned Nonproductive hours:* The vaction, holiday, education leave, sick leave, etc. hours are budgeted for the coming year.
6. *Productive and nonproductive time:* To aid in the planning process, a graph is used to show head and assistant head nurses how the level of forecasted patient days—and therefore the staffing requirements—are expected to move up and down during the year. Productive time is the time spent on the job in patient care, administration of the unit, conferences, educational activities, and orientation.

Only steps seven and eight are concerned with nonlabor expenses:

7. *Supplies and services:* Here the supplies and purchased services for the year are budgeted.
8. *Capital budget:* This is where the expected capital investments for the coming year are figured into the budget.

These eight steps result in a total budget package which goes to the director of nursing services for review. Upon his or her preliminary acceptance of this budget, it is sent to the accounting department, where the forecasted patient days are turned into expected revenue. The budgeted productive and nonproductive time is extended into dollars, as are the costs for supplies and services and other operating expenses that will be allocated to a given nursing unit for the coming year. A pro-forma operating statement is then returned to the director of nursing for review, with the head nurse. When the director of nursing and the head nurse accept the budget, it is returned to the accounting department and forwarded with the rest of the hospital budgets to administration and the Board of Directors.


## LABOR BUDGET ORIENTATION

At El Camino Hospital, we have found that involvement of the head and assistant head nurse is a key element in the planning and budgeting process. To prepare nurses for this process, orientation sessions are held for those key people involved in budget preparation. We will now take a look at the steps and the people that make the process work efficiently.

An important resource for the head nurse is the budget coordinator. Budgeting is viewed as an ongoing process, and the coordinator has the responsibility of preparing and making available the information head nurses need to make intelligent budgetary decisions. This responsibility includes documenting any changes that take place in the unit's fiscal operations and helping to prepare any required remedial action plans.

The budget coordinator must educate and orient the nursing staff to the complex budgetary systems because few nurses have been trained in this management function. The coordinator conducts a series of two-hour sessions with each unit's head nurse and assistant head nurses. On many units, staff nurses as well participate in these orientation sessions. Inclusion of assistant head nurses and staff nurses serves to motivate and educate greater numbers of the staff to this process. This tends to support the team approach to unit monetary goals and to bring awareness of these goals to the staff-nurse level. It encourages participation and interest in aspects of hospital management which were never before considered by staff nurses.


### The First Session

At the first orientation session, the budget coordinator reviews the following information:

- Staffing philosophy concept used in a decentralized system
- The clinical-unit staffing policy
- Unit time schedules
- Time-card documentation

In addition, the nurses learn about the feedback systems used for analysis of activity and performance. The following reports are generated every pay period for their use:

- Labor analysis report
- Nursing productivity cost center report
- Labor distribution
- Patient dependency categorization report
- Labor performance report

Documentation is stressed as the foundation of all budgeting, and these reports provide the data necessary for monitoring the unit's activities, for retrospective problem solving, and for determining changes or trends in patient activities. Each report is discussed in detail.

*Labor Analysis Report.* This report is generated automatically from the payroll time-card data. It shows for the total hospital all productive hours worked (both regular time and overtime) and nonproductive hours by categories of paid time off. Each one of these categories of time is shown by employee job code in hours, both for the current pay period and year-to-date.

*Nursing Productivity Cost Center Report.* The budget coordinator extracts from the labor analysis report this summary of each nursing unit's productivity by cost center. It is a valuable collection of data for both the director of nursing and the head nurse. It gives them an overall picture of how the nursing units are doing, individually and collectively.

*Labor Distribution Report.* This contains the same information as the labor analysis report, except it indicates individuals by name rather than by job code. It shows the head nurse who is employed on the unit and how much coded time has been utilized every pay period.

*Patient Dependency Categorization Report.* This is a summary of documented required hours for patient care, divided by actual hours worked in providing that care. It shows all categories of patients rated from one to four by shift (patient dependency system). The unit's goal for this report should be 100-percent utilization, although the range indicated on the report is from 90-110 percent. This document is issued through the management engineering department every two weeks (equivalent to the hospital's pay period).

*Labor Performance Report.* A summary of a unit's earned standard hours divided by the actual hours worked for all cost centers, this report includes information about the unit's overall goal by pay period and year-to-date figures.

**The Second Session**

At the second orientation meeting the budget coordinator explains the four cost centers necessary for the preparation of a unit budget:

- Administration
- New training
- Education
- Patient care

These four cost centers reflect the activity on a nursing unit. They also allow for the differentiation of productive time spent in direct patient care from productive time spent in managing the unit and educating the personnel.

*Administration.* Coded to this cost center is the time spent by the head nurse and unit personnel in managing the nursing unit. Some examples of how the time is used include coaching staff, completing performance appraisals, attending meetings, updating and revising unit policies and procedures, unit planning, and nursing research. The head nurse shares the administrative hours with assistant head nurses and staff nurses, depending on management responsibilities delegated to them.

*New Training.* Orientation of new personnel and orientation of current nursing staff to a new area of responsibility is coded to new training. Also allocated to the NT cost center are the hours spent by nurses who are serving as preceptors to new employees.

*Education.* Nursing unit educational conferences, in-house educational programs and independent learning time spent by nurses in the hospital's learning center are coded to the education cost center.

*Patient Care.* All nursing time spent in patient care is coded to this cost center. Also coded here is the time worked by the unit secretaries.

Hours are estimated for each of these cost centers. The hours for new training, education, administrative and patient care cost centers differ according to the kind of unit and will be negotiated between the head nurse and the director of nursing during actual budget sessions. The nursing unit's overall goal is a summary of the hours and negotiated goals of the four cost centers.

**The Third Session and the Follow-up**

A third orientation session is spent reviewing and discussing the information presented at the first two meetings. The nurses by this time have had the opportunity to absorb and apply what was learned at the first two sessions.

Following these orientation sessions the staff nurse who attended often serves as a resource to fellow nurses, answering their questions about budget, productivity, and staffing. Often it is difficult for staff nurses to understand the importance of productivity goals,—how they are determined, how they are achieved, and exactly how they relate to staffing. This staff-nurse resource, therefore, is extremely valuable in assisting his or her peers to understand the budget process.

The nursing units vary in the intensity with which staff nurses are involved in the budgeting process. Our experience indicates that those areas where the majority of staff is involved and educated are more supportive and under-standing of the system and their role in attaining the goals.

At the actual budget session, time is spent in a careful analysis of each individual unit. An effort is made to identify any changes or differences from past years. Such differences may include any changes in the average length of stay and in the types of patients being cared for. The staff turnover rate and hiring practices will also be examined. The budget coordinator seeks to show how (or if) these changes may affect the coming year's budget, and works with unit personnel and the director of nurses to identify which differences or changes may make the unit's current goals difficult or impossible to achieve.

When making out the labor budget, the basic question to be answered by any given nursing unit is, *How much staff is too much, and how much staff is too little?*

## THE LABOR BUDGET PROCESS AT WORK

To better understand how the labor budget system works, let's look in on a typical budget session. Shirley, the head nurse of 2-East, a 34-bed general surgical unit, is meeting with the director of nursing, the budget coordinator and the management engineer. Also present are Shirley's assistant head nurses and a staff nurse. They are animatedly discussing last year's productiv-ity and the expected census levels and patient mix for the coming year. Shirely's current productivity goal for 2-East is 94 percent. The director of nursing would like a new productivity goal of 95 percent set for the coming year. The director's rationale for a productivity goal is based on the nursing unit's history of past performance and its trend, known future events that would affect productivity, and overall nursing service and hospital goals with respect to the next fiscal year's productivity.

On examining Shirley's year-to-date productivity, the director is pleased to find that 2-East has attained a 94.5-percent productivity. The unit has exceeded its own expectation. Shireley and her staff look for reasons, and they find two: First, the hospital began a transportation service last year, decreasing the amount of time nurses were required to be away from trans-porting patients throughout the hospital. This has particularly helped to increase the productivity of the day and evening nurses. Second, the hospital instituted an exchange cart-supply program, automatically stocking the nurs-ing units every 24 hours with supplies and equipment that previously had to be ordered for each patient or on a weekly order basis. Freeing the nurses from constant reordering, checking inventory, and searching for supplies has allowed them to devote more productive hours to their prime responsibility—the patient.

Shirley and her staff agree to the 95-percent productivity goal. They have reviewed the census forecast and have found a typical yearly pattern has been predicted. There is no forecast for any changes in the patient mix or the major/minor surgery mix on 2-East. The forecast makes good sense to the nurses. It is agreed that the new goal of 95 percent is both realistic and achievable. It will become one of Shirley's written unit objectives for the coming year.

---

### 2-EAST PATIENT DAY FORECAST
### FISCAL YEAR

| Accounting Period:* | 1 | 2 | 3 | 4 | 5 | 6 | 7 |
|---|---|---|---|---|---|---|---|
| Patient Days: | 750 | 750 | 780 | 740 | 740 | 750 | 740 |
| Accounting Period: | 8 | 9 | 10 | 11 | 12 | 13 | TOTAL |
| Patient Days: | 790 | 775 | 775 | 740 | 770 | 740 | 9,795 |

---

*Accounting Period = 28-day period consisting of 4 complete weeks with 13 accounting periods per fiscal year.*

---

### Budgeting Labor

Shirley's next task is to determine the number of staff that she needs to take care of the forecasted patient census. She uses a budget worksheet to determine the total number of full-time equivalents (FTEs) that are needed for 2-East, based on her productivity goal and anticipated census. She takes into account the hours of patient care needed, the vacation and holidays that this staff will accumulate during the coming year, the average amount of sick time used, and other significant factors that will require additional coverage—e.g., education, orientation, administrative time, and paid educational leave. Upon completion of the budget worksheet, Shirley has determined the number of FTEs that she needs to staff 2-East. She compares the number with her current number of employees and determines the number of people she needs to hire for each shift, if any. Two questions have been answered: *(1)How much staff should Shirley hire to care for these patients? (2) How much staff should be scheduled on day shift, evening shift, and night shift?*

|  |  |
|---|---|
| Day shift: | 13.0 FTEs |
| Evening shift: | 9.8 FTEs |
| Night shift: | 5.6 FTEs |
| Department total: | 28.4 FTEs required for patient care |

Now Shirley must ascertain how much staff should be assigned to each shift each day of the week. The management engineer will review with Shirley last year's historical census pattern (Exhibit 4–2). The census by day of the week has been kept and graphed by the management engineer and will help to determine the most frequent census level for each day of the week for the coming year. The recommended weekly staffing schedule worksheet (Exhibit 4–3) is used to translate the expected census level each day into the required staff for each shift each day. This information is then transferred to a recommended weekly time schedule (Exhibit 4–4) which represets a midpoint or core-staffing guide per shift per day for the coming year. Also on this form is the full-time (FT) and part-time (PT) staffing mix by classification (RN, LVN, and NA) required to attain the recommended schedule and provide for the every-other-weekend-off scheduling requirements. By scheduling a minimum of core staff per shift per day, Shirley will be scheduling the most likely complement of staff required to meet the patient-care needs for each shift each day of the week. Of course, the actual needs may dictate deviation from the core-staffing pattern based on higher- or lower-than-usual patient census and/or acuity levels. (The hospital utilizes variable staffing techniques in all nursing units which base the actual staffing on the nurses' assessment of each patient's care requirements.)

Another question—*How much will the staffing needs vary by day of the week?*—has been answered. Next year's core staffing pattern for 2-East is:

## SCHEDULED STAFF BY SHIFT BY DAY

| Day: | Sun | Mon | Tue | Wed | Thu | Fri | Sat |
|---|---|---|---|---|---|---|---|
| Day Shift | 6 | 7 | 7–8 | 8 | 8 | 8 | 6–7 |
| Evening Shift | 5 | 6 | 7 | 7 | 6–7 | 6 | 5 |
| Night Shift | 2–3 | 3–4 | 4 | 4 | 4 | 3–4 | 2–3 |

Shirley has one remaining question: *How much and when can vacation time be scheduled?* In order to answer this question, Shirley and her staff review the forecasted workload (converted to productive patient care hours). The workload is distributed across the year by accounting period and reflects the amount of staff necessary for patient care. The difference between the FTEs required for patient care (28.4) and the total FTEs (29.05) reflects when and how much vacation time may be scheduled; thus the forecasted census is translated into the required number of nursing care hours by pay period.

The result is the expected number of patient care hours required by shift each pay period across the year to take care of the expected patient census. Shirley adds this information on a staff planning graph, which shows how the workload varies by pay period across the year. The graph (Exhibit 4–5) also

**Exhibit 4-2.    Historical Census Pattern**

### HISTORICAL CENSUS PATTERN

NURSING UNIT ____*2·EAST*____          DATA PERIOD _____

|  | SUN | MON | TUE | WED | THU | FRI | SAT | ALL DAYS |
|---|---|---|---|---|---|---|---|---|
| TOTAL CENSUS | 1247 | 1480 | 1392 | 1599 | 1367 | 1393 | 1152 | 10,030 |
| NUMBER OF DAYS | 51 | 52 | 52 | 52 | 52 | 52 | 51 | 362 |
| AVERAGE | 24.45 | 28.46 | 30.61 | 30.75 | 30.13 | 26.79 | 22.59 | 27 |
| VARIANCE | 12.48 | 15.44 | 7.47 | 6.11 | 9.34 | 11.17 | 10.32 | |
| STD. DEVIATION $\sqrt{\text{VARIANCE}}$ | 3.53 | 3.93 | 2.73 | 2.47 | 3.05 | 3.34 | 3.21 | |

### AVERAGE CENSUS BY DAY OF THE WEEK

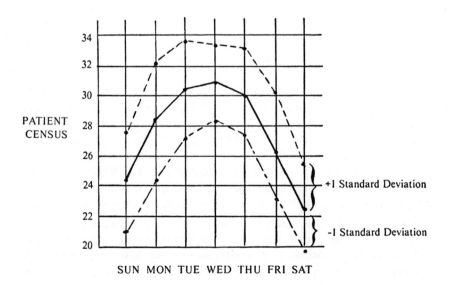

PATIENT CENSUS

+1 Standard Deviation

-1 Standard Deviation

SUN MON TUE WED THU FRI SAT

Exhibit 4-3.  Recommended Weekly Staffing Schedule Worksheet

## RECOMMENDED WEEKLY STAFFING
## SCHEDULE WORKSHEET

UNIT ____Z-EAST____          CENSUS DATA PERIOD _____

|  | AVE. CENSUS | H.P.P.D. x CENSUS | HOURS/ DAY | STAFF (÷ by 3) | DAY x 44% | PM x 36% | NITE x 20% |
|---|---|---|---|---|---|---|---|
| SUNDAY | 23.88 | 5.09 | 121.55 | 15.19 | 6.68 | 5.47 | 3.04 |
| MONDAY | 27.79 | 5.09 | 141.45 | 17.68 | 7.78 | 6.36 | 3.54 |
| TUESDAY | 29.89 | 5.09 | 152.14 | 19.62 | 8.37 | 6.85 | 3.80 |
| WEDNESDAY | 30.03 | 5.09 | 152.85 | 19.11 | 8.41 | 6.88 | 3.82 |
| THURSDAY | 29.42 | 5.09 | 149.75 | 18.72 | 8.24 | 6.74 | 3.74 |
| FRIDAY | 26.16 | 5.09 | 133.15 | 16.64 | 7.32 | 5.99 | 3.33 |
| SATURDAY | 22.06 | 5.09 | 112.29 | 14.04 | 6.18 | 5.05 | 2.81 |
| TOTAL FTE'S: (SUM ÷ 5 SHIFTS/FTE) | | | | | 10.6 | 3.7 | 4.8 |

shows from the budget worksheet the number of FTEs that are available for patient care as well as to provide coverage for administrative, education, orientation, vacation, holiday, and average sick time. The difference between the staff available and the expected patient-care requirements is the time available to give the staff their vacations, and holidays as well as coverage for these other functions. The graph displays these variables by amount and time of year. Thus the last question —*How much and when can vacation time be scheduled?*—has been answered.

Then the vacation and holiday time is scheduled on a personnel budget-by-position form (Exhibit 4-6). On this form the number of hours to be worked by each classificaion of staff on each shift each pay period in patient care is shown. The sum of these hours equals the required number of nursing-care hours by pay period. The number of hours expected to be used in administrative, education, and orientation time across the year is also shown. The planned vacation time from the staff planning graph along with average sick

**Exhibit 4-4.   Recommended Weekly Time Schedule**

UNIT ___*2-EAST*___         **BUDGET YEAR** _____

*Recommended Time Schedule*

| | SUN | MON | TUE | WED | THU | FRI | SAT | *Full-Time/Part-Time Mix* | | FT | PT |
|---|---|---|---|---|---|---|---|---|---|---|---|
| AVE. CENSUS | 24 | 28 | 30 | 30 | 29 | 26 | 22 | | | | |
| DAYS | 6 | 7 | 7/8 | 8 | 8 | 8 | 6/7 | DAYS | RN | 5 | 4 |
| | | | | | | | | | LVN | | 2 |
| | | | | | | | | | NA | 2 | |
| | | | | | | | | | CUS | 1 | |
| | | | | | | | | | | | |
| PMS | 5 | 6 | 7 | 7 | 6/7 | 6 | 5 | PMS | RN | 4 | 5 |
| | | | | | | | | | LVN | | |
| | | | | | | | | | NA | | 2 |
| | | | | | | | | | CUS | | 1 |
| | | | | | | | | | | | |
| NITES | 2/3 | 3/4 | 4 | 4 | 4 | 3/4 | 2/3 | NITES | RN | 2 | 2 |
| | | | | | | | | | LVN | 1 | |
| | | | | | | | | | NA | 1 | |
| | | | | | | | | | CUS | | |
| | | | | | | | | | | | |

**Exhibit 4-5. Staff Planning Graph**

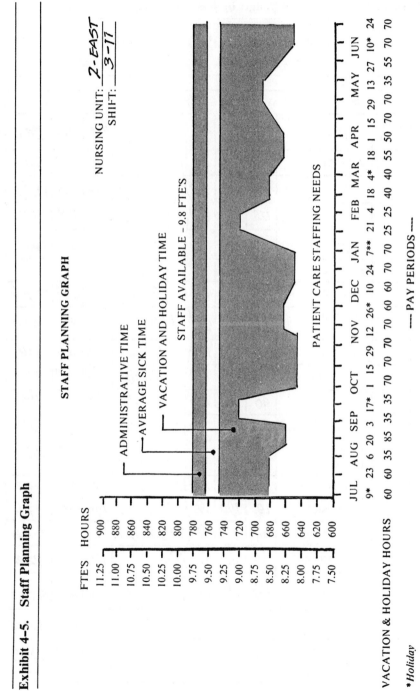

STAFF PLANNING GRAPH

NURSING UNIT: 2-EAST
SHIFT: 3-11

*Holiday

**Exhibit 4–6.   Personnel Budget by Position**

## PERSONNEL BUDGET BY POSITION

DEPARTMENT ___2-EAST___        SHIFT ___3-11___

| JOB CODE | POSITION | 1978 ———— PAY PERIOD ENDING | | | | 1979 | | | | |
|---|---|---|---|---|---|---|---|---|---|---|
| | | 7/8 | 7/22 | 8/5 | 8/... | 5/12 | 5/26 | 4/9 | 4/23 | TOTAL |
| | AHN/CHG | 112 | 112 | 112 | | 112 | 112 | 112 | 112 | 2912 |
| | RN II | 383 | 383 | 360 | | 372 | 374 | 374 | 379 | 10,042 |
| | NA | 128 | 128 | 128 | | 128 | 128 | 128 | 128 | 3326 |
| | CUS | 64 | 64 | 64 | | 64 | 64 | 64 | 64 | 1664 |
| | | | | | | | | | | |
| | TOTAL PT. CARE | 687 | 687 | 664 | | 6.78 | 6.78 | 6.78 | 6.79 | 17,946 |
| | PT. CARE FTE ÷ 30 | 8.6 | 8.6 | 8.3 | | 8.5 | 8.5 | 8.5 | 8.5 | 8.68 |
| | ADMINISTRAT. | 16.0 | 16.0 | 16.0 | | 16.0 | 16.0 | 16.0 | 16.0 | 416 |
| | ORIENTATION | 16.0 | 16.0 | 16.0 | | 16.0 | 16.0 | 16.0 | 16.0 | 416 |
| | EDUCATION | 40 | 40 | 40 | 4 | 40 | 40 | 40 | | 104 |
| | TOT PROD HRS. | 723 | 723 | 700 | 70.. | 714 | 714 | 714 | | 18,392 |
| | BIRTHDAY & FLOAT HOLID. | 59 | 59 | 58 | 59 | 5.9 | 5.9 | 5.9 | | 153.4 |
| | HOLIDAY (7) | 384 | 384 | | | | 384 | 384 | | 499 |
| | AVER. SICK | 190 | 190 | 190 | | 196 | 190 | 190 | 196 | 494 |
| | EDUC. LEAVE | 5.7 | 5.7 | 5.7 | | 5.7 | 5.7 | 5.7 | 5.7 | 148.8 |
| | VACATIONS | 64 | 64 | 80 | | | | 84 | 84 | 728 |
| | TOTAL NON-PRODUCT HRS. | 133 | 133 | 110.5 | | | 93 | 93 | 93 | 3023.2 |
| | TOTAL PD. HRS. | 857 | 856 | 811 | 7 | 807 | 807 | 801 | | 30925 |
| | TOTAL FTE'S ÷ 30 | 10.7 | 10.7 | 10.1 | | | 10.1 | 10.1 | 10.7 | 10.05 |

time and paid educational leave is also indicated. The labor portion of 2-East's budget is complete.

During the budget meeting, Shirley has formulated her plan for the coming year. She now knows how much staff is too much and how much staff is too little, in the process the following questions have been answered:

- What should the productivity goal be for 2-East for the coming year? (A goal of 95 percent was established.)
- How many patients can the nursing unit expect during the coming year? (Patient days expected for 2-East total 9795. January through March are expected to be high-census months; August through December, except for September, are low-census months.)
- How much staff should Shirley hire to care for these patients? (Budgeted FTEs = 29.05 for productive and nonproductive time.)
- How much staff should be hired for day shift, evening shift and night shift? (Day shift = 13.0 FTEs; evening shift = 9.8 FTEs; and night shift = 5.6 FTEs.)
- How much will the staffing needs vary by day or by week?
- How much and when can vacation time be scheduled?

These questions have been answered by reviewing the census forecast and determining the high-and low-census months.

Shirley's core staffing pattern for the next year has been established. The minimum personnel required to meet core staffing is set and Shirley has guidelines for when and how much vacation time to schedule during the year. The hours budgeted for education and orientation of new employees to the unit are added to the complement of personnel hired to the unit. The resulting total budgeted FTEs for 2-East then is:

Day shift     = 13.26 FTEs
Evening shift = 10.06 FTEs
Night shift   =  5.73 FTEs

TOTAL         = 29.05 FTEs

Completion of the budget worksheet gives Shirley and her assistant head nurses the recommended number of FTEs for the coming year. This is the number of FTEs they will use in planning their annual labor budget. Although the labor budget is more complex, the remaining components of the budget are no less important. These include allocation of supplies and services and capital expenditure.

*Budget Worksheet.* The budget worksheet is an important tool in this budgeting process. Using the budget worksheet and the budget parameters for 2-East, a productivity goal of 95 percent, a labor standard of 4.84 nursing hours per patient day (HPPD), and a patient-day forecast of 9795, the necessary complement of staff is determined. Then, by accounting for the vacation and holidays that the staff will accumulate, the average amount of sick time used and other significant factors that require nursing staff coverage, the number of full-time equivalents that Shirley needs to staff 2-East for the coming fiscal year is calculated.

We have seen how the productivity goal and forecasted patient days are determined. The third parameter, 2-East's labor standard, was based upon work done by the management engineering department and nursing service, using traditional time-study methods. Over time, patient-care parameters that affect the labor standard have been identified and quantified. The labor standard would be lowered, for example, by the introduction of a computerized medical information system. Parameters that would raise the labor standard might include the decreasing length of patient stay in the hospital, an aging patient population, and the opening of an ambulatory surgicare center resulting in a higher mix of major surgical patients on the general acute surgical units.

On the budget worksheet for 2-East (Exhibit 4–7) the 9795 patient days are turned into average daily patient days. The nursing hours per patient day (HPPD) are 5.09, which is equivalent to the labor standard of 4.84 HPPD at a 95-percent productivity goal. The average daily patient days are multiplied by 5.09 HPPD, resulting in an average daily productive hour requirement for patient care of 136.92 hours. These average daily productive hours are converted into the number of staff, and the number of FTEs required is 23.97 (or 24).

The average daily productive hours by shift are then determined. Here the average daily productive hours of 136.92 are spread across or allocated to the three various shifts. They are allocated on a percentage basis with the day shift receiving 44 percent of the total hours, evening shift 36 percent, and night shift 20 percent. These percentages are based upon management-engineering work done at the hospital; they reflect typical industry standards for hospitals. The average hours per day for each shift are then turned into the staff required for each day and the number of full-time equivalents required for each shift; days require 10.54, evenings 8.62 and nights 4.79 FTEs. These are the full-time equivalents required to take care of the average daily census for 9795 patient days per year at 4.84 HPPD and with a goal of 95-percent productivity.

Staff requirements for 2-East to cover the number of holidays, education leave and vacation time that these twenty-four FTEs will accrue must be determined. These needs are considered under nonproductive time coverage. Using the day shift as an example, the seven holidays that occur at specific times throughout the year are shown as 56 hours times 10.54 FTEs = 590.2 hours. For educational leave the projected number of FTE RNs on the day shift, 7.4, times 24 hours of educational leave per RN results in 177.6 hours of educational leave budgeted. The day-shift personnel also accrue some 32.8

**Exhibit 4-7. Budget Worksheet.**

## BUDGET WORKSHEET

NURSING UNIT: ___2 EAST___   BUDGET PERIOD: _____

| ANNUAL PATIENT DAYS: *9795* |
|---|

AVERAGE DAILY PATIENT DAYS: *26.9* @ *5.09* H.P.D. *4.84* @ *95% Goal*

AVERAGE DAILY PRODUCTIVE HOURS *136.9* ÷ 8 = *17.12* STAFF x 1.4 = *23%* FTE's

### AVERAGE DAILY PRODUCTIVE HOURS BY SHIFT

|  | HOURS | STAFF | | FTE's |
|---|---|---|---|---|
| DAY | *44* : *60.24* ÷ 8 | *7.83* | x 1.4 | *10.54* |
| EVE | *36* : *49.29* ÷ 8 | *6.16* | x 1.4 | *8.63* |
| NITE | *20* : *29.38* ÷ 8 | *3.42* | x 1.4 | *4.79* |

### NON-PRODUCTIVE TIME COVERAGE

| SHIFT | HOLIDAYS | | E.L. | VACATION | FTE'S |
|---|---|---|---|---|---|
| | HR/PROD FTE FTE HRS | HR/PROD FTE FTE HRS | HR/PROD FTE FTE HRS | HR/ WK WK HRS | HR/ HRS FTE FTE |
| DAY | 56 x *10.54* = *590.2* | 16 x *10.54* = *168.6* | 24 x *7.4* = *177.6* | *32.8* x 40 = *1312* | *2245.4*/2000 = *1.12* |
| EVE | 56 x *8.62* = *482.7* | 16 x *8.62* = *137.9* | 24 x *6.2* = *148.8* | *18.2* x 40 = *728* | *1497.4*/2000 = *.75* |
| NITE | 56 x *4.79* = *268.2* | 16 x *4.79* = *76.6* | 24 x *3.2* = *76.8* | *16.4* x 40 = *656* | *1077.6*/2000 = *.59* |

### FTE'S

|  | DAY | EVENING | NITE |
|---|---|---|---|
| 1. PRODUCTIVE | *10.54* | *8.62* | *4.79* |
| 2. VACATION/ HOLIDAY/EL | *1.12* | *.75* | *.54* |
| 3. AVE. SICK TIME | *.475* | *.237* | *.147* |
| 4. ADMINISTRATIVE | *.87* | *.2* | *.1* |
| 5. | | | |
| 6. TOTAL FTE'S HIRED  (1 thru 5) | *13.0* | *9.8* | *5.6* |
| 7. EDUCATION | *.11* | *.05* | *.05* |
| 8. ORIENTATION | *.145* | *.2* | *.1* |
| 9. | | | |
| TOTAL BUDGETED FTE'S  (1 thru 4 -7 and 8) | *13.26* | *10.06* | *5.73* |

| DEPARTMENT TOTAL BUDGETED FTE'S | *29.05* |
|---|---|

weeks of vacation; multiplying this times 40 hours results in 1312 hours of vacation budgeted for the coming year. The resultant nonproductive time amounts to 2,248.4 hours; dividing this by 2000 hours, estimating some two weeks off during the year for holidays and sick leave, results in 1.12 FTEs needed to provide nonproductive time coverage for the 10.5 FTEs involved in patient care. These various elements for each shift are summed up in the lower portion of the budget worksheet.

The sum of patient care hours for each shift, vacation/holiday and educational leave for each shift, average sick time for each shift, and budgeted administrative time results in the total number of FTEs hired to 2-East for the next fiscal year:

Day shift     = 13.0 FTEs
Evening shift = 9.8 FTEs
Night shift   = 5.6 FTEs

## SUPPLIES AND SERVICES BUDGET

The supplies and services budget also relies upon the patient-day forecast. The use of medical and nonmedical supplies is based upon the forecasted patient days for the coming year. The average cost of medical and nonmedical supplies is determined from the preceding year's expense plus the expected inflationary increases.

Purchased services are based on historical information and reflect any service contracts particular to that unit. The input for this budget is primarily from accounting data that the head nurse reviews. She may make changes based on anticipated changes in the type and amount of supplies required for the coming year. The major tool in figuring the supplies and services budget is the nonlabor expense worksheet, a copy of which is shown in Exhibit 4–8.

## CAPITAL BUDGET

As head nurse, Shirley must also budget for each item costing over $250 that she plans to purchase within the next three years. These expenses are figured on a capital expenditure worksheet (Exhibit 4–9). After conferring with the assistant head nurses and the director of nursing, Shirley will plan for the purchase of new equipment and/or the replacement of existing equipment. The capital expenditure worksheet includes a description of the item, the importance and urgency of its acquisition, and other requested information. Head nurses are required to indicate in which quarter the equipment should be purchased and to specify annual equipment needs for the following two years. The capital expenditure worksheets are used by the purchasing agent and hospital administration in developing a capital expenditure budget for the next three years.

# Exhibit 4-8. Nonlabor Expense Worksheet

| Accounting Period | 1 | 2 | 3 | 4 | 5 | 6 | 7 | 8 | 9 | 10 | 11 | 12 | 13 | TOTAL |
|---|---|---|---|---|---|---|---|---|---|---|---|---|---|---|
| 1. UNITS OF SERVICE: | | | | | | | | | | | | | | |
| *Supply Expense* | | | | | | | | | | | | | | |
| 2. Average Effective Rate—Drugs, Food | | | | | | | | | | | | | | |
| 3. *DRUGS—FOOD—LINEN EXPENSE* *(Line 1 x Line 2)* | | | | | | | | | | | | | | |
| 4. Floor Nourishments (Estimate) | | | | | | | | | | | | | | |
| 5. Average Effective Rate—Medical Supplies | | | | | | | | | | | | | | |
| 6. *MEDICAL SUPPLY EXPENSE* *(Line 1 x Line 5)* | | | | | | | | | | | | | | |
| 7. Average Effective Rate—Nonmedical Supplies | | | | | | | | | | | | | | |
| 8. *NONMEDICAL SUPPLY EXPENSE* *(Line 1 x Line 7)* | | | | | | | | | | | | | | |
| 9. Maintenance—Repair Supplies | | | | | | | | | | | | | | |
| 10. *TOTAL SUPPLY EXPENSE* | | | | | | | | | | | | | | |
| *FEES & PURCHASED SERVICES* | | | | | | | | | | | | | | |
| 11. Professional Fees—Physicians | | | | | | | | | | | | | | |
| 12. Professional Fees—Administrative | | | | | | | | | | | | | | |
| 13. Purchased Services (Estimate) | | | | | | | | | | | | | | |
| 14. Equipment Repair & Maintenance Services (Est.) | | | | | | | | | | | | | | |
| 15. *TOTAL FEES & SERVICES* | | | | | | | | | | | | | | |
| *GENERAL & ADMINISTRATIVE* | | | | | | | | | | | | | | |
| 16. Depreciation—Equipment (Assets) | | | | | | | | | | | | | | |
| 17. Leases and Rentals | | | | | | | | | | | | | | |
| 18. Utilities | | | | | | | | | | | | | | |
| 19. Education  Tuition—Travel | | | | | | | | | | | | | | |
| 20. Other General & Administrative | | | | | | | | | | | | | | |
| 21. *TOTAL GENERAL & ADMINISTRATIVE* | | | | | | | | | | | | | | |
| 22. *GRAND TOTAL NONLABOR EXPENSES* | | | | | | | | | | | | | | |

**Exhibit 4–9.   Capital Expenditure Worksheet**

| COLUMN # | 1 | 2 | 3 | 4 | 5 | 6 | 7 | 8 | | 9 | | | | 10 | 11 |
|---|---|---|---|---|---|---|---|---|---|---|---|---|---|---|---|
| | | | | | | | | EST'D COST | | ACQUISITION PERIOD (5) | | | | DEPARTMENTAL | ADMINISTRATIVE |
| ITEM | (1) DESCRIPTION OF ITEM | (2) PRIORITY | ADDITION | REPLACEMENT | (3) DISPOSAL | (4) RENOVATE | QUANTITY | EACH $ | TOTAL $ | 1st Qtr. | 2nd Qtr. | 3rd Qtr. | 4th Qtr. | COMMENTS (JUSTIFICATION) | COMMENTS/ APPROVAL |
| 1. | | | | | | | | | | | | | | | |
| 2. | | | | | | | | | | | | | | | |
| 3. | | | | | | | | | | | | | | | |
| 8. | | | | | | | | | | | | | | | |
| 9. | | | | | | | | | | | | | | | |
| 10. | | | | | | | | | | | | | | | |

(1) List in order within year, priority, disposals last.

(2) Priority:
a. Required for accreditation and licensure.
b. Cost reduction.
c. Required for objective.
d. Desired for other reasons (specify).

(3) Disposal:
T. Trade-in
S. Sale
R. Retire & store
D. Transfer for other use
J. Scrap

(4) Renovate: Repair & extend useful life.
(5) Acquisition: Indicate *month* desired in column.

REMARKS: _____
_____

## TOTAL BUDGET

Shirley and her assistant head nurses have completed the budgeting process for the coming year. They recognize that the ultimate success of the detailed plan they helped develop is dependent upon all the nurses who work on 2-East. Staff-nurse involvement at the budget and orientation sessions significantly increases their knowledge and sense of responsibility towards implementing their unit's budget. Another positive aspect is that these nurses become aware of how their unit's budget affects the hospital's total budgetary operations.

This same process must be carried out by the budget coordinator in fifteen other nursing units before the deadline for submission of the total nursing-service budget. When this is done, all sixteen budgets are sent to the hospital accounting department to be combined into a complete departmental budget. The complete budget then goes to the hospital's administrative office for review and incorporation into the final hospital budget. This in turn is submitted to the Board of Directors for their final approval.

From this review, it should be clear that the nursing component for the overall hospital budget includes expected revenue, productive and nonproductive time, supplies, capital expenditures, and much other information, all of which has been prepared with or by the head nurses of the hospital's sixteen units. Valuable resources are provided by many support people, particularly the budget coordinator, management engineer, and accountants.

In preparing their budgets, the head nurses carry out an exercise in management. Further, they become familiar with the fiscal aspects of their responsibility and learn how to plan for the coming year. Although they receive a great deal of help from the budget coordinator, the ultimate decision as to how they will manage their part of the total hospital budget throughout the next fiscal year is theirs.

### Budget Surveillance

The completion of the budgetary process, however, does not signal the end of the budget-planning activities in a decentralized nursing service. Ongoing surveillance of the budget reminds nurses that everything that happens in a nursing unit during a year has its effect not only on that unit's budget, but also on the fiscal operations of the entire nursing service and on the ultimate provision of cost-effective patient care.

Several tools are available to help head nurses monitor the financial condition of their units. They receive a nurse-utilization report each two-week period, allowing them to review their labor productivity by shift and as a total department. Other reports show which categories of individuals are reporting time to the unit each shift. Thus head nurses are able to see the

**Exhibit 4-10.   Remedial Action Plan Summary.**

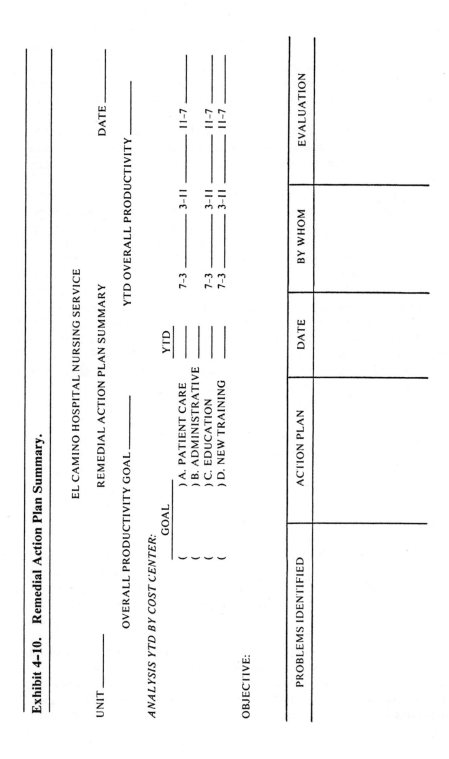

names of the actual staff members who are charging time by shift and by cost center. A unit operating statement for each accounting period shows actual revenues and expenses, compares these figures with budgeted figures, and accumulates them into year-to-date figures. At two-week intervals the budget coordinator reexamines what is happening to each unit's operation. Timely and accurate feedback is essential. Where deficiencies appear, the coordinator will point them out to the head nurse of the unit involved. Together they will investigate and look for reasons why the deficiency is occurring. Remedial action reports may be initiated when it's clear that the reasons are preventable and require follow-up measures. The identified problems are entered on a remedial action plan summary (Exhibit 4–10) along with the reasons for their occurrence and the head nurse's action plan for dealing with them. Also noted is the person responsible for the action plan and the date it was initiated.

Each month the budget coordinator meets with the head nurses in their complex meeting. At this time their remedial action plan is reviewed in group discussion and evaluated as to success. Head nurses give one another a wealth of support as they draw from mutual experience in problem solving. The budget coordinator makes recommendations and assists in remedial action planning—but, as always, the decision on what will be done rests with the individual head nurse. Accountability is therefore derived through feedback, not from an administrative power base. This is a critical component in keeping the philosophy and structure of a decentralized organization alive and well.

Content for this chapter was taken in part from "Planning and Budgets, Magic or Math" by John Fleming, June 1978. Published in *Maintaining Cost Effectiveness,* Elsie Schmied (ed.), Nursing Resource Books, Inc., Wakefield, Mass., pp. 229–246.

# 5

## *Quality Assurance: Collaborating for Patient Care*

On 3-West there's a meeting in progress. The unit's head nurse and four staff nurses have gathered to discuss the criteria by which the quality of patient care is to be judged. Half a dozen years ago they would have had little reason to consider this issue; today they are being asked to set the standards for the level of their own performance.

The discussion at the meeting is lively. Jennifer, the head nurse, is the quietest of the group, allowing the staff nurses free discussion. The quality assurance coordinator, Gail, starts things off and acts as an advisor. She's concerned about the recurring problem of patient falls. Before the meeting Gail recommended that the group read an article, a study showing that an initial assessment can pinpoint which patients are prone to falls. This, Gail believes, may make it possible to work out corrective-action criteria before a fall takes place.

Gail asks the group to give her direction in incorporating the criteria into an audit form that she is preparing. The form should determine whether a proper assessment for falls has been done and if the proper preventative measures have been taken.

Some of the questions she asks include these:

- What should be noted in the initial assessment?
- What preventative actions should be taken?
- How should they be documented?

The group responds with enthusiasm to Gail's request for information and answers. Together they agree on a set of criteria for the problem. Some criteria are debated and discarded because they don't seem practical. Some are rejected outright as unrealistic. Soon a series of practical, workable ideas begins to emerge from the discussion. Some of the criteria are approved conditionally. They will be tried. If they prove unwieldy or impractical, they will be revised or eliminated before the next audit of the unit. Good, workable criteria will be retained.

The nurses leave the meeting with a positive feeling. They have been involved in the development process and are now able to discuss with other members of their unit and with the rest of the hospital nursing staff the problem of how to deal with patient falls. The resulting combination of information and feedback will be gathered and considered. It will become a set of permanent criteria to be added to the present concurrent audit form. Eventually, too, there will be sufficient statistical information to make comparisons and to see if, indeed, falls in the hospital have decreased.

## DEVELOPING DECENTRALIZED QUALITY ASSURANCE

This process of audit may seem slow but it is quickening. Gradually, nurses are learning to incorporate new documentations and procedures into their practice. As a problem in care is identified, the group that sets the criteria by which it is judged and corrected is the one most directly involved in rendering that care. For example, criteria for falls will be developed from the medical, surgical, and orthopedic units of the hospital. Criteria for preoperative teaching techniques, on the other hand, will be developed by nurses on the surgical units. Literature is researched, feedback from educational programs is integrated, and nursing standards are reviewed. Objective literature is integrated with practical knowledge and skill in order to set criteria with a solid theoretical base and practical application.

This approach is a considerable change from that used in the past. Criteria are set with the knowledge gained from expert clinicians—the nurses at the bedside. Because they are performing the daily nursing care, staff and head nurses have the expertise necessary to develop the most practical way to audit and improve care. When their suggestions are accepted and implemented, it proves to the nursing staff that their views *do* make a difference.

Under the traditional system of nursing organization, it's unlikely that nurses would have had a chance to do this. The traditional system tended to view the question of individual and group performance as a personal expression of the director of nursing services and his or her supervisors. Usually the measurement of the quality of nursing care was made solely from chart audits. These were checked to see that nursing tasks were adequately noted in the patient's record. No attempt was made to ask a patient questions or to evaluate the patient's progress toward wellness.

As concern about the measurement of the quality of care became more pressing, the emphasis in the assessment of that quality shifted to outcome criteria. The system for developing criteria also shifted. We began to use the nurses whose care would be audited to determine how it should be performed.

We believe in this practice. Involving the people closest to the problem has made the recognition and solutions of problems more effective.

The meeting on 3-West and many others like it have been the result. These sessions have allowed staff and head nurses the chance to decide for themselves which criteria are most important and to participate in the process of developing a system of quality assurance.

The problem, of course, has not simply been one of agreement. It also has been necessary to make criteria into a coherent, ongoing program of quality assurance. And even before this, we have had to define what we mean by these words.

## Defining Quality Assurance

At El Camino, we define quality assurance as *a program to make certain that the quality of nursing care remains at a consistently high level.*

Similar definitions have been given by others. Here are some examples of what they are saying:

"Activities done to determine the extent to which a phenomenon fulfills certain values, and activities done to assure changes in practice which will fulfill the highest levels of values."[1]

"Quality Assurance has as its central goal making certain that care practices will produce good patient outcomes."[2]

"Quality assurance . . . refers to the accountability of health personnel for the quality of care they provide."[3]

Whatever its definition, quality assurance is not a new issue, either in nursing or in other areas of health care. Maintaining the quality of nursing care—indeed, maintaining all medical care at a high level—has always been important. What has become increasingly evident, however, is the rising demand from others that this be so.

The demand has come from many places. Government is one. More and more, government is demanding to know how the money it provides for health care is spent. The Joint Commission on the Accreditation of Hospitals is another. Its standards have become the rule for the operation of many phases of hospital care, not only for nursing but for all facets of the health-care picture. The consumers themselves represent a third. Spurred by the growth of the consumer movement, they want an active voice in determining how they are treated when they are sick. Decentralization has helped us to respond to these pressures.

## The Quality Assurance Coordinator

The position of quality assurance coordinator was created in our nursing department at the time of the decentralization process. A former supervisor with audit experience volunteered to oversee the efforts to establish a quality assurance program. She presented a proposal to management council and obtained approval to begin the program. It became her responsibility not only to put the criteria developed by nursing units into some kind of a workable system, but also to develop the forms, methods of gathering information, and uses for such data.

In the process it became clear that the quality assurance coordinator could not function as either a police officer or a spy. The new quality assurance program was intended to be cooperative. It was not to be imposed on the nursing structure, but generated from within. It rested squarely on common consent and enthusiasm, especially from staff and head nurses.

The nursing staff still remained accoutable to the director of nurses, as did the quality assurance coordinator. The intent of the program was to increase participation, to draw from the organization, to use the inverted pyramid that is our picture of how nursing service should work. The quality assurance coordinator is shown on the organizational chart in a line position to the director and in a staff position to the complexes, a resource to be utilized by the line personnel and accountable to the director.

## Developing Criteria

The quality assurance coordinator's first task was to develop criteria to be used in measuring the quality of care. The audit process consists of criteria development, measurement, reporting, evaluation, corrective action, reevaluation and reporting. When establishing clinical criteria, there are several points to consider:

- Criteria must be specific enough so that they allow only one interpretation.
- Criteria must be concise and written in short, clear phrases; they must be understandable.
- Criteria must be clinically sound so as to reflect current clinical practice and judgment.
- Criteria must be achievable and should require reasonable performance behaviors.

The question of how to develop these criteria was answered at El Camino Hospital by utilizing the nurses whose care would be audited.

In 1973, groups of staff nurses were gathered together to develop nursing standards for common nursing conditions in their various specialities. These criteria or standards were published in the form of *Standard Nursing Care Plans.* [4] The standard care plans are written in such a way that the indicators representing satisfactory progress are clearly stated as "expected outcomes." The basis for the first and ongoing audit criteria for El Camino Hospital was developed from these expected outcomes. Outcome criteria indicate the end result of patient care: a measurable change in the state of patient health. This care-planning system is used currently at El Camino Hospital and has been incorporated in the computerized medical information system.

## AUDITING

Patient care can be assessed in two ways: retrospective review and concurrent review. Retrospective review at El Camino is jointly performed by medical and nursing staff as a patient-care audit. The review includes all assessment mechanisms that are utilized to review care following the patient's discharge. Areas of concern in patient care are identified by various medical and nursing committees and reported to the Medical Audit Committee, which includes the quality assurance coordinator in its membership. The committee selects the diagnosis associated with that concern. Physicians develop medical criteria and the quality assurance coordinator works with the nursing staff to develop nursing criteria. Medical-records personnel use these criteria to compile the audit data. The results of the audit are reviewed before the Medical Audit Committee by physicians and nursing personnel. The committee reviews the results and makes recommendations to the appropriate medical committee or physician. Frequently, both physician and nursing actions are necessary to remedy a deficit. The quality assurance coordinator reviews the results with the nursing staff for remedial action of identified deficiencies. This joint-audit procedure has enhanced collaboration between physicians and nurses in improving the quality of patient care at El Camino Hospital.

Retrospective audit at El Camino is performed through closed-chart audits, post-care questionnaires, patient interviews and staff conferences. A look at some of the retrospective audit tools may be helpful. Exhibit 5-1 shows criteria examples and results. A remedial action form is shown in Exhibit 5-2, and a post-care questionnaire appears as Exhibit 5-3. These tools were designed to give the nursing staff feedback on the quality of patient care based on documentation of outcomes.

Concurrent review can be performed through open-chart audits, patient interviews, unit visits, and staff reviews. A prime advantage of concurrent review is that the audit findings may be acted upon promptly and have an immediate impact on patient care. The concurrent review tools for El Camino are included: Exhibit 5-4 shows a total nursing care evaluation form, and Exhibit 5-5 outlines the audit procedure. The scoring procedure appears as Exhibit 5-6, and a sample total evaluation report is shown in Exhibit 5-7. Exhibit 5-8 gives an example of a concurrent remedial action report. These tools were designed to give the nursing staff feedback on a quarterly basis and their quality scores on patient care and care planning. Concurrent audits are carried out at random on a specific unit by the quality assurance coordinator.

**Exhibit 5-1.    Criteria Examples and Results**

*TOTAL HIP REPLACEMENT* (NURSING CRITERIA)

|  |  | CRIT. | EXC. | VAR. |
|---|---|---|---|---|
| 1. | Patient and/or family received pre-op. teaching and he/she can verbalize what to expect regarding pre- and post-op. procedures. | 100% | 81 | 0 | 19 |
| 2. | Afebrile<br>A.  Discharge with M.D. aware of temp. elevation. | 100% | 98 | 1 | 2 |
| 3. | Well-healed wound<br>A.  M.D. aware; discharge AMA | 100% | 95 | 5 | 0 |
| 4. | Ambulatory—crutches and/or walker<br>A.  M.D. notified of pain on discharge | 100% | 96 | 3 | 1 |
| 5. | Free of surgical pain<br>A.  M.D. notified of pain on discharge | 100% | 96 | 4 | 0 |
| 6. | Patient and/or significant others demonstrate understanding of activity limitations | 100% | 72 | 0 | 28 |
| 7. | Voiding quantity sufficient (q.s.) | 100% | 100 | 0 | 0 |
| 8. | B.M. at least 3 days before discharge | 100% | 97 | 0 | 3 |
| 9. | No falls | 100% | 100 | 0 | 0 |

Perhaps an example will show the kinds of information sought. Here is an excerpt from a concurrent audit form, in this case a section devoted to hydration and fluid balance.

1. Fluid at bedside (NPO/NA)
2. IV fluid
   a. Date and time?
   b. Correct fluid?
   c. Correct amount and rate?
   d. Medication labeled?
   e. IV site red and tender?
   f. Tubing w/extension secured?
   g. IV site labeled with date, needle size, and RN?
   h. IV tubing and dressing changed q 24°?

To each of these questions the quality assurance coordinator seeks a "yes" or "no" or "not applicable" answer. Other sections of the form include questions about skin integrity, ventilation, musculoskeletal function, nutri-

---

**Exhibit 5-2.    El Camino Hospital Remedial Action Plan**

---

DATE:    *January, 1981 through June, 1981*
DIAGNOSIS/PROCEDURE:    *Total Hip Replacement*

1.  STATEMENT OF DEFICIENCY:

   *Patient pre-op teaching 100% (actual 81%) (19% deficit)*
   *Patient demonstrates understanding of activity limitations 100% (actual 72%)  (28% deficit)*

2.  (A) SOURCE OF DEFICIENCY:

   GROUP ____*X*_____
   INDIVIDUAL _____
   INSTITUTION _____

   (B) REASONS FOR DEFICIENCY:

   KNOWLEDGE ____*X*_____
   PERFORMANCE _____
      LACK OF FEEDBACK _____
      TASK INTERFERENCE _____
      APATHY _____
      OTHER _____

3.  SHORT TERM PROGRAM OBJECTIVES & DATE FOR COMPLETION:

4.  REMEDIAL ACTION PROGRAM:

   *Review audit findings with nursing staff.*
   *Mini conference on audit criteria and review charting philosophy for ECH.*

5.  PERSON RESPONSIBLE FOR REMEDIAL PROGRAM:

   *Head nurse*

6.  CONCURRENT MONITORING (if needed):

   *Random sample of charts weekly—next 4-6 weeks.*

7.  DATE FOR REAUDIT:

   *(If random sample results favorable, none required.)*

REPORT RECEIVED BY: _____HEAD NURSE                    DATE _____


REPORT RECEIVED BY: _____ DIRECTOR OF NURSING    DATE _____


REPORT RECEIVED BY: _____ QUALITY ASSURANCE
                                             COORDINATOR                DATE_____

## Exhibit 5-3.    El Camino Hospital Nursing Service
## M-S-O Post Care Questionnaire

*At our hospital, we are interested in providing you with the best possible care. In this questionnaire, we want to know your reactions to your recent hospital experience.*
*ALL ANSWERS REMAIN COMPLETELY ANONYMOUS AND CONFIDENTIAL.*
*Please complete this brief questionnaire and return it in the enclosed envelope. Thank you for your assistance.*

*Sincerely,*

*Nursing Audit Coordinator*
*Quality Assurance*

After each statement please check the answer that most closely fits your recent hospital experience.

1.  How were you initially received in the Admitting Department?
    Friendly _____    Unfriendly _____  Indifferent _____
2.  Were you kept waiting to have your lab work done?    Yes _____ No _____  NA _____
3.  Were you kept waiting to have your X-ray work done?  Yes _____ No _____  NA _____
4.  Were you escorted to your room by hospital personnel? Yes _____ No _____ NA _____
5.  How was your initial reception on the unit?  Friendly ___ Unfriendly ___ Indifferent ___
6.  Did you understand how to use the call button and other equipment?
    Yes _____        No _____
7.  Were your meals prepared tastefully?    Yes _____        No _____
8.  Were you visited by the dietician?    Yes _____      No _____
9.  Was your room kept clean?  Yes _____        No _____        NA _____
10. Were you asked to do your own care even though you didn't feel up to it?
    Yes _____    No _____        NA _____
11. Did you always receive assistance to relieve pain promptly?
    Yes _____    No _____    NA _____
12. Did you know what to expect regarding treatments, procedures and care?
    Yes _____    No _____
13. Were you able to identify the persons caring for you?  Yes _____      No _____
14. Were you allowed to have family or friends you needed near you?
    Yes _____    No _____
15. Did you feel confident about the nurses caring for you? Yes _____  No _____
16. Did you feel that you were allowed privacy when you needed it?  Yes _____ No _____
17. Did you receive the emotional support you needed while you were in the hospital?
    Yes _____    No _____    NA _____
18. Did the nurses take time to listen when you had concerns or ideas about your care?
    Yes _____    No _____    NA _____
19. Did anyone teach you what you needed to know to resume your own care at home?
    Yes _____    No _____    Doctor_____    Nurse_____
20. Did you participate in a teaching program in any of the following? Yes _____ No _____
    Which one?    Diabetes ____ Coronary Rehab _____ Colostomy ____ IV ____
    If so were they helpful?    Yes _____        No _____        NA _____
21. Please recommend one change that you feel would improve the services offered to patients at El Camino Hospital:

    _____

    _____

    Other comments/suggestions:

    _____

---

**Exhibit 5–4.   El Camino Hospital Evaluation of Total Nursing Care**

---

DATE _____ UNIT _____          Patient Label
DIAGNOSIS _____
TRANSFERRED FROM _____ DATE TRANSFERRED ____
EVALUATION DONE BY _____

### I.  PHYSICAL NEEDS
A. Skin Integrity

| Patient Care | YES | NO | NA | Care Plan/Documentation | YES | NO | NA |
|---|---|---|---|---|---|---|---|
| 1. Clean and dry: | ___ | ___ | ___ | I.  Problems Identified: | ___ | ___ | ___ |
| 2. Skin Dry? | ___ | ___ | ___ | II.  Nursing orders re: | | | |
| 3. Odor? | ___ | ___ | ___ | a. Skin Care | ___ | ___ | ___ |
| 4. Reddened? | ___ | ___ | ___ | b. Decubiti prevention | ___ | ___ | ___ |
| 5. Decubiti? | ___ | ___ | ___ | c. Decubiti care | ___ | ___ | ___ |
| 6. Pressure areas apparent? | ___ | ___ | ___ | III.  Plan in current format | ___ | ___ | ___ |
| 7. Rash? | ___ | ___ | ___ | IV.  E/O reflected in N/N | ___ | ___ | ___ |

B. Hydration and Fluid Balance

| Patient Care | YES | NO | NA | Care Plan/Documentation | YES | NO | NA |
|---|---|---|---|---|---|---|---|
| 1. Fluid at bedside (NPO/NA) | ___ | ___ | ___ | I.  Problem Identified: | ___ | ___ | ___ |
| 2. IV fluid: | | | | II.  NO regarding: | | | |
| a. Date and time? | ___ | ___ | ___ | a. Limit fluids | ___ | ___ | ___ |
| b. Correct fluid? | ___ | ___ | ___ | b. Encourage fluids | ___ | ___ | ___ |
| c. Correct amt. & rate? | ___ | ___ | ___ | c. IV fluids | ___ | ___ | ___ |
| d. Medication labeled? | ___ | ___ | ___ | III.  Plan in current format | ___ | ___ | ___ |
| e. IV red or tender? | ___ | ___ | ___ | IV.  E/O reflected in N/N | ___ | ___ | ___ |
| f. Tubing w/extension secured | ___ | ___ | ___ | | | | |
| g. IV site labeled with date, needle size & RN? | ___ | ___ | ___ | | | | |
| h. IV tubing & dressing changed: | ___ | ___ | ___ | | | | |
| i. Rotation of sites? | ___ | ___ | ___ | | | | |
| 3. Hydration: | | | | | | | |
| a. Limitation? | ___ | ___ | ___ | | | | |
| b. Push? | ___ | ___ | ___ | | | | |
| 4. Heparin lock? | ___ | ___ | ___ | | | | |
| a. Site labeled with date, needle size and RN? | ___ | ___ | ___ | | | | |

**Exhibit 5-4.    *(continued)*[1]**

C. Respiratory Status

| Patient Care | YES | NO | NA | Care Plan/Documentation | YES | NO | NA |
|---|---|---|---|---|---|---|---|
| 1. Patient turns regularly? | — | — | — | I. Problem Identified | — | — | — |
| 2. Patient supports chest, op. site when coughing? | — | — | — | II. NO regarding: a. Positioning | — | — | — |
| 3. Problems with breathing a. Preventive | — | — | — | b. Turning regularly c. Deep breathing | — | — | — |
| 4. Tracheostomy: a. Needs suctioning? | — | — | — | d. Coughing e. Trach care | — | — | — |
| b. Approp. equipment? | — | — | — | f. Pt. teaching | — | — | — |
| c. Humidification? | — | — | — | g. Chest tube routine | — | — | — |
| 5. Chest tubes patent? | — | — | — | h. Comm. method | — | — | — |
| a. Emergency clamp? | — | — | — | III. Plan in current format | — | — | — |
| 6. Suction equipment? | — | — | — | IV. E/O reflected in N.N. | — | — | — |
| 7. Respiratory supportive equipment? | — | — | — | | | | |

D. Musculoskeletal Function

| Patient Care | YES | NO | NA | Care Plan/Documentation | YES | NO | NA |
|---|---|---|---|---|---|---|---|
| 1. Activity as ordered? | — | — | — | I. Problem Identified? | — | — | — |
| 2. Muscle conditioning? | — | — | — | II. Nursing orders regarding: | | | |
| 3. Corrective equipment? | — | — | — | 1. Activity (type and amount)? | — | — | — |
| 4. Needs assistance? | — | — | — | 2. Muscle conditioning? | — | — | — |
| 5. Body in alignment? | — | — | — | 3. Corrective equipment identified? | — | — | — |
| 6. Patient knows activity Rx? | — | — | — | 4. Number of people needed to assist patient? | — | — | — |
| | | | | 5. Plan in correct form? | — | — | — |
| | | | | 6. E/O reflected in N.N.? | — | — | — |

**Exhibit 5-4.**    *(continued)*

E. Dietary

| Patient Care | YES | NO | NA | Care Plan/Documentation | YES | NO | NA |
|---|---|---|---|---|---|---|---|
| 1. Satisfied with diet? | — | | — | 1. Nursing/dietary orders re: | — | | — |
| 2. Patient knows diet | | | | 1. Food preferences? | | | |
| Rx/reason? | — | | — | 2. Food allergies? | | | |
| 3. Patient knows food | | | | 3. Special diet/feeding | | | |
| allowed? | — | | — | needs ID? | — | | — |
| 4. Patient assisted w/meals? | — | | — | | | | |

F. Elimination

| Patient Care | YES | NO | NA | Care Plan/Documentation | YES | NO | NA |
|---|---|---|---|---|---|---|---|
| 1. Patient feels elimination | | | | 1. Nursing orders regarding: | | | |
| adequate: | — | | — | 1. Bladder problems? | | | |
| a. Bowels? | — | | — | a. Plan in correct form? | — | | — |
| b. Bladder? | — | | — | b. E/O reflected | | | |
| 2. Patient with draining | | | | in N.N.? | — | | — |
| systems? | — | | — | 2. Bowel problems? | | | |
| a. Drainage bag secured | | | | a. Plan in correct form? | — | | — |
| properly? | — | | — | b. E/O reflected | | | |
| b. Tubing straight and | | | | in N.N.? | | | |
| kink-free? | — | | — | 3. Type of catheter: | | | |
| c. Catheter & equip. | | | | a. Date inserted? | — | | — |
| clean? | — | | — | b. Date changed? | — | | — |
| 3. Patient incontinent: | — | | — | c. Size? | — | | — |
| a. Clean and dry? | — | | — | 4. Catheter care? | — | | — |
| 4. N.G. tube patent or | | | | 5. Bowel function | | | |
| clamped? | — | | — | recorded? | — | | — |
| | | | | 6. Irrigation procedure | | | |
| | | | | identified? | — | | — |
| | | | | 7. Status of N.G. tube? | — | | — |

*A complete copy of this form appears in the Appendix of this book.*

---

**Exhibit 5-5.   Audit Procedure**

---

### EL CAMINO HOSPITAL
### NURSING SERVICE

*CONCURRENT AUDIT TOOL PROCEDURE*

1.  Random selection of patients.
2.  Number of patients audited is determined by size of unit, i.e., 34-bed unit—8 patients will be sampled. (1/4 of the patients).
3.  Questions are formulated from the tool by using the left hand column.
4.  If there is a problem identified on the left hand column, then the problem should be identified on the care plan, using the right hand column as a guide.
5.  Unit audits are conducted within 8 hours and results with feedback are given to Head Nurses within 24 hours.
6.  Audits are conducted on each nursing unit every three months.
7.  Nursing units are always unaware of when the concurrent audit will be done.

---

tional status, elimination, hygiene, physical comfort, rest and sleep, and hospital safety.

The section of the form relating to psycho-social needs includes spaces for information on the patient's sense of security and his or her need for any spiritual support. Information gathered about therapeutic and rehabilitative needs examines self-care and discharge planning. The hospital safety questions deal with varied aspects of patient care and some legal requirements. They are meant to raise awareness as well as to determine the nurse's individual competence.

**Audit Results**

Each head nurse has goals and objectives relative to concurrent and retrospective auditing. These goals and objectives are mutually identified and agreed upon with the director of nursing services. Audit scores in many ways reflect how these goals and objectives have been met. A head nurse may have an average composite audit score of 85 percent and decide mutually with the director to set a goal of 90 percent for the next year. The head nurse will probably post this unit goal and discuss its significance and implications with the staff. There will be emphasis on the unit's attainment of that goal. In a year's time the new unit score will be determined and part of the head nurse's performance evaluation will be based on how well he or she accomplished the goal of 90 percent.

What other effects do audit reports have? To a great extent this depends on

---

**Exhibit 5-6.    Scoring Procedure**

---

### EL CAMINO HOSPITAL
### NURSING SERVICE

## *EVALUATION OF TOTAL NURSING CARE SCORING METHOD*

1.  The evaluation will be scored in the following categories (attachment) A.
2.  Determine a percentage score for each heading under I-A, I-B, I-C, II-A, II-B, and II-C. The percentage score is
$$= \frac{\text{number of correct answers}}{\text{number of applicable questions.}}$$
3.  Determine the percentage score for I-A, I-B, I-C, II-A, II-B, and II-C by multiplying the percentage scores under each heading (item 2) by its weighted value and summing these results. (Weighted value is decided by the nursing staff.)
4.  Determine the patient care score by multiplying the scores for I-A, I-B, and I-C by their respective weighted percentages and sum the results.
5.  Determine the care planning score by following the instructions in item 4 using the scores for II-A, II-B, and II-C.
6.  The total score is the sum of I and II (items 5 & 6) divided by two (2).

---

the perceived causes of the deficiencies noted, but in any case the emphasis on using the information they contain is positive.

Possible solutions are noted and discussed by the quality assurance coordinator with the head nurse and the staff nurses of the unit being surveyed. If the deficiency is because of a lack of knowledge, then obviously steps must be taken to ensure that such knowledge is gathered and disseminated to those who need it. If the deficiency is due to a lack of equipment, then efforts must be made to obtain the necessary equipment and put it to use. If there is a deficiency resulting from inadequate staff, the head nurse has an obligation to identify the specific need and follow through with such appropriate action as hiring additional staff or changing staffing patterns.

At some point in the discussion of problem areas, a method of reevaluating and reexamining the problem is jointly discussed and agreed to by the quality assurance coordinator and the head nurse of the specific unit under audit. When deficiencies in care are found on a unit, concurrent random sampling may be started. Depending on the random sampling results and the seriousness of the deficiency, a date for reaudit may or may not be set.

The coordinator presents data from audits to the Board of Directors on a routine basis. This input keeps them informed of the level of care consumers are receiving at El Camino Hospital. Audit data is one part of the myriad of information that the Board of Directors uses when making recommendations about broad aspects of hospital policy concerning patient care.

---

**Exhibit 5-7.    Total Evaluation Report**

---

## EL CAMINO HOSPITAL
## NURSING SERVICE

| | |
|---|---|
| PURPOSE: | Evaluation of total nursing care |
| UNIT: | 2-North |
| CENSUS: | 27 |
| SAMPLE SIZE: | 7 |
| STUDY PERIOD: | August 1978 |
| OVERALL QUALITY | (Pt. care & Care planning) |
| Complete: | 89% |
| Patient Care: | 94.5% |
| Care Planning: | 84% |

    I.  PATIENT CARE:
        A.  Physical needs—98%
        B.  Psycho-social needs—91%
        C.  Teaching needs—100%
   II.  CARE PLANNING:
        A.  Physical needs—98%
        B.  Phycho-social needs—73%
        C.  Teaching needs—81%
 III.  Hospital Safety—85%

---

## Incident Reports

Incident reports at El Camino Hospital are similar to those at other hospitals, in most respects. They are required in any situation where the hospital might incur liability because of the action or lack of action by hospital personnel. Exhibit 5-9 is a computer printout of a typical incident report.

A unique feature of the El Camino incident report requires the nurse involved to write remedial actions. This is intended to place accountability and is a critical step in the quality assurance process. The report describes the situation and the incident and any steps which may be required to ensure that it does not happen again. This action places responsibility on the nurse involved. In the process of writing the remedial action report, the responsible nurse develops a sense of control over his or her own practice. The end result of this accountability can be a greater sense of self-worth and increased job satisfaction. That is why the report must be assigned to the nurse responsible for the patient involved in the incident: any other way of handling the requirement would defeat the effectiveness of the process. Incident report summaries (see Exhibit 5-10) are sent to the units every quarter. Incident reports are also reviewed quarterly with the director of nursing services, and objectives and goals are defined.

---

**Exhibit 5-8.    Concurrent Remedial Action Report**

---

### EL CAMINO HOSPITAL
### NURSING SERVICE

REPORTING DEFICITS & PLAN FOR CORRECTIVE ACTION
CONCURRENT AUDIT

DATE    8/78                                           UNIT    2-North

I.    Identified Areas for Improvement:

1. N.C.P. – Psycho-social needs.

2. N.C.P. - Teaching needs.

3. Hospital safety.

II.    Remedial Action Program:
*Action*

1. NCP –Psycho-social needs: Assess patient on admission as to feelings about hospitalization and document.

2. NCP – Teaching needs—Document discharge teaching.

3. Hospital safety—Review monthly disaster protocols.

III.    Person Responsible for Remedial Program:
Nancy Nurse

IV.    Goals:

1. NCP – Increase score to 80%.

2. NCP – Increase score to 85%.

3. Hospital safety—Increase score to 90% by next audit.

---

Report rec'd by _____ , Head Nurse
Report rec'd by _____ , Director of Nursing
Report rec'd by _____ , Nursing Audit Coord.

---

## BENEFITS OF QUALITY ASSURANCE

It is important to understand that the system measures unit performance in a way not possible under authoritarian nursing. In effect, the head nurse and her staff nurses are setting realistic goals for themselves and are assisting the entire service in reaching a common quality of care.

Failure to achieve the nursing-unit goal does not result in punitive reaction from the director of nursing services, but instead produces a positive set of

---

**Exhibit 5-9.    Incident Report**

---

### EL CAMINO HOSPITAL

11/30/81          10:26 AM

PT INCIDENT— **DOE, JOHN**                                                                    PG-1
DATE 11/30/79                    TIME 11:15 PM                    EMP# 03421
BED RAILS UP  YES                                    BED POSITION LOW __
SAFETY BELT USED  NO __                            PT RATIONAL  YES
ACTIVITY B.R.P. WITH__HELP _____
DR SMITH _____ NOTIF AT 11:30 PM
BY JANE BROWN__R.N. _____ UNIT—4 WEST__
NAME & ADD OF 2 PEOPLE FAMILIAR W DETAILS
1. MARY__JONES__R.N.__E.C.H.  ˙_____

---

2. JOHN GREEN__N.A.__E.C.H.  _____

---

NARC/SEDATIVES GIVEN 12 HRS PRIOR TO INCIDENT, DOSE & TIME—
DALMANE 15 MGM. PO AT 9PM.

PT ACCOUNT OF INCIDENT—PT STATES HE WANTED TO GO TO BATHROOM
AND DIDN'T WANT TO BOTHER ANYONE.

NURSE ACCOUNT (INCLUDE EXACT LOCAL)—PT FOUND ON FLOOR NEAR
BATHROOM. PT CONSCIOUS. ASSISTED BACK TO BED. VITAL SIGNS NORMAL.
MOVES ALL EXTREMITIES. ABRASION ON FOREHEAD OVER LEFT EYE.

REMEDIAL PLAN—PT. INSTRUCTED TO USE CALL BELL WHEN HE WANTS TO
GET OUT OF BED. WILL MAKE A NOTE ON CARE PLAN TO REINFORCE USE OF
CALL LIGHT AS PT. IS RELUCTANT TO ASK FOR HELP.

---

steps to remedy the problems revealed by the auditing procedure. To this end head nurses often ask the quality assurance coordinator to sit in on meetings at which deficiencies are discussed. The coordinator's helpful insight into problems has proven valuable in developing remedies. Other benefits of quality assurance include these:

- Meeting the public's need for accountability in nursing care.
- A better understanding of patient-care patterns in the hospital.
- A better discernment of where there is a need for documentation.
- Encouragement of coordination and communication of patient care planning with other health-care disciplines.
- Methods of improving patient care, both in the short and long term.
- Location of general deficiencies in hospital policies and procedures.

---

**Exhibit 5-10.    Incident Report Summary**

---

## EL CAMINO HOSPITAL NURSING SERVICE

SUMMARY OF INCIDENT REPORTS FROM _____THROUGH_____

| UNIT | SHIFT | MED | I.V. | FALLS |
|------|-------|-----|------|-------|
| 4 East | 7-3 | 2 | 2 | 2 |
| | 3-11 | 2 | 1 | 3 |
| | 11-7 | 1 | 1 | 3 |
| | | | | |
| | | | | |
| TOTAL | | 5 | 4 | 8 |

1 patient went AMA.
1 patient lost his glasses.
1 patient spilled hot tea on arm —first-degree burn.

Compared to last quarter, all incidents are down.

---

- A more meaningful way for health-care providers to participate in and achieve career growth.
- A better method of allowing health-care providers to establish standards of patient care.
- A better outlook for the patient.

### Further Responsibilities of the Quality Assurance Coordinator

The quality assurance coordinator has a number of responsibilities beyond auditing and incident report review. One such responsibility is to log all litigation in progress against the hospital and monitor its outcome, particularly any outcome that may involve the nursing service.

The quality assurance coordinator's position provides an improved avenue

---

**Exhibit 5-11.    Poster about Quality Assurance**

---

# QUALITY ASSURANCE ALERT!

Statistics gathered from the recent quarterly Incident Reports have shown evidence of a marked increase in patient falls.

The Quality Assurance Committee is having a difficult time identifying the reasons for this increase. We are asking for your suggestions and ideas in an effort to help us reduce the number of falls.

Please contact Nancy Smith, Quality Assurance Coordinator, with any suggestions you might have.

Some safety reminders we can ask ourselves are:

1.   Are patients reminded to call for assistance when needed for ambulation?
2.   Are beds and side rails checked for correct position?
3.   Are restraints being used when they are necessary?

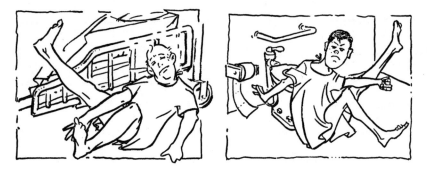

*Adapted from drawing by John A. Smith*

---

of communication, not only for the nursing staff, but also for the patients. The coordinator interacts with many different groups throughout the hospital, often using humorous or informative posters to call attention to special problems. Exhibits 5-11 and 5-12 provide some examples of these. The quality assurance coordinator has ongoing rapport with hospital administration and physicians.

Because of contact with patients during the auditing process, the quality assurance coordinator is more aware of patient complaints and may be able to deal with them from a different perspective than nurses on the unit. The ability to move between units, the director of nursing services, and the hospital administration provides a valuable liaison between patients and the hospital itself.

The quality assurance coordinator also has educational responsibilities. By providing an ongoing audit, this individual is able to teach auditing as a

---

**Exhibit 5-12.   Poster about Quality Assurance**

---

# QUALITY
# ASSURANCE
# ALERT

Quality Assurance involves both evaluation and improvement actions in patient care.
What part do Incident Reports play in Quality Assurance?
They identify areas in patient care that need improvement.
In the past three (3) months there were seventy-two (72) medication errors. Each one
was a violation of one or more of the "Five Rights":

      1.  Right patient
      2.  Right drug
      3.  Right dose
      4.  Right time
      5.  Right route

Ask yourself if you are remembering those five rights?
- Are you waiting for the initial dose if ordered from pharmacy? (Pharmacists check
  for drug incompatabilities and drug allergies.)
- Are you checking for new doctor's orders prior to giving meds?
- Are you using *Nursing Care Plan* or *Meds Due List* for bedside check against
  patient's I.D. band?

                Quality Assurance Committee

---

process to other members of the staff. Auditing data, gathered in a planned
and objective manner, allows for better staff care planning. Improved charting by the nurses—the result of continuing audits—gives the nursing service
data useful in improving the quality of care. Audit has been used to emphasize
the need for nursing care plans and to document improved performance in
this area. It can serve the same function in other departments of the hospital.

The quality assurance coordinator participates in Executive Committee
meetings of the nursing staff, sits on Management Council sessions, listens
and responds to patient and family problems, helps to track down patients'
lost valuables, relieves other coordinators when required, and is a member of
a number of important nursing and medical staff committees, including
Medical Audit, Chart, Quality Assessment, Concurrent Review, and Infection Control.

## SUMMARY

How has quality assurance been received by members of the nursing staff? It would be untrue to say that it has been universally and immediately accepted. In some units, participation by staff nurses remains to be completely accomplished. In others, it has been a part of nursing care planning and is now integrated into the day-to-day operation of the unit.

Enthusiasm for the program is growing. A thoughtful staff nurse, who also has been an assistant head nurse, believes one of its immediate benefits has been the increased ability of nurses to work with physicians on an equal basis:

"There's a generally positive feeling about it," she says. "What amazes me are the day-to-day things I see. I participate more with physicians now. There is a lot more input from them. I think we are better able to speak up and to provide input than we were under the previous system. When you take responsibility, you feel other people should be more responsible for what they are doing."

The growing understanding of the need for collaboration with the entire hospital health team is one of the greatest benefits of the new emphasis on quality assurance. Obviously, nurses do not work in a vacuum. Much of what they hope to accomplish in outcomes of quality patient care is dependent on other practitioners within the hospital. Dietitians, lab techonologists, x-ray personnel, pharmacists, and the myriad of others who give direct and indirect patient care are all involved.

The end result of quality patient care depends on the good performance of these ancillary departments in their own specialized areas of function. Undoubtedly the model developed by the nursing quality assurance coordinator will be used by other departments to audit performance. When this goal is accomplished, the total patient care will be monitored and a much more accurate picture of the quality of care will be available. This comprehensive audit also will meet the requirements of the 1980 JACH accreditation manual for hospitals, which provides for audit of all clinical departments, disciplines and individual practitioners.

The final common goal of all hospital personnel, of course is the provision of superior quality patient care. This is the end result of all nursing, all medical, all work activities in the hospital.

In an atmosphere where criteria for care are formed by those most responsible for its delivery, it is possible for all health care workers to make valid contributions. The ultimate criteria from such an effort will be reflected in what happens to our patients. And that, we believe, is the best measure of quality assurance there is.

# REFERENCES

1. N. Lang, *A Model for Quality Assurance in Nursing*, p. 11. Unpublished doctoral dissertation, Marquette University, 1974.
2. M.G.Mayers, R.B. Norby, A.B. Watson, *Quality Assurance for Patient Care: Nursing Perspectives* (New York: Appleton-Century-Crofts, 1977), p. 3.
3. B. Brown, "Quality Assurance," *Nursing Administrator* Q.1:V, Spring 1977.
4. Marlene Mayers and El Camino Hospital, *Standard Nursing Care Plans*, Vols. I, II, and III (Palo Alto, CA: K.P. Co. Medical Systems, 1974, 1975, 1977).

# 6

# Staff Development: Enhancing Professional Skills

Under El Camino Hospital's decentralized nursing system a department of education and training provides ongoing staff development programs designed to maintain the highest quality standards in patient care. We consider our staff development unique in that it offers the following combination of features:

- Managerial training for head nurses and assistant head nurses, nursing coordinators, and staff development instructors through the establishment of a Management and Organizational Development program (MOD).
- Clinically oriented staff development instructors who provide educational support on all three shifts.
- Coaching and validation of skills at the bedside by staff development instructors.
- Individualized, self-paced learning supported by our own learning center.
- Development and support of staff nurses as preceptors and resource nurses.

## THE IMPORTANCE OF STAFF DEVELOPMENT

At El Camino Hospital, staff development has been made a separate department. Those nurses who, under centralized nursing, were a part of nursing inservice education now are designated staff development instructors in the new department of education and training (see Exhibit 6–1).

As such, they function as one of the principal support groups within decentralized nursing, organized to assist the nurse at the bedside. Together with the nursing coordinators, the staff development instructors work to improve the efficiency and ease of the staff nurse's job. Coordinators assist with management support; staff development instructors provide educational

---

**Exhibit 6-1.   Department Chart**

---

EL CAMINO HOSPITAL
DEPARTMENT OF EDUCATION AND TRAINING

*DIRECTOR*--------------------Secretary

*Nursing Staff Development*

One Maternal-Child-Health instructor
One Dialysis Unit instructor
Two Critical-Care instructors
Two Medical-Surgical-Orthopedics instructors  days
One Medical-Surgical-Orthopedics instructor evenings
One Medical-Surgical-Orthopedics instructor nights

*Management
and Organizational
Development*
One trainer

*General Education*
One instructor

*Audiovisual Services*
Director
One technician

*Health Education*
Director--------------------Secretary (2)
Three instructors

---

support. This educational support includes all available resources—equipment, materials, and instruction.

The individual responsibilities of the staff development instructors are diverse, but all are expected to do assessment, planning, implementation, and evaluation of the educational function for nursing service. Individual teaching style and creativity is encouraged. The way in which each instructor functions will, however, be determined in part by the size and needs of the nursing complex she or he serves. At El Camino Hospital, staff development instructors are assigned to each of the nursing complexes within nursing service and provide educational support on a regular basis to all three shifts.

Staff development instructors coordinate the orientation of new employees and assist them in adapting to performance expectations and hospital routines. Instructors are often asked to chair nursing committees and task forces, to do research on clinical issues, and to spearhead the development of new nursing procedures.

As a clinical role model and expert resource, staff development instructors must maintain and update their skills and knowledge. Therefore special emphasis is placed on reading professional journals, on attending workshops and seminars, and on assisting in direct patient care.

The latter task is of special importance, for it provides the instructor with current "hands-on" experience which can be passed on to other nurses. Instructors are expected to spend a part of each week on nursing units, coaching and validating nursing skills of staff nurses and generally assisting with patient-care decisions.

Instructors are involved in many professional activities within the community. They teach courses at local colleges and universities; they act as liaison between the hospital and community by chairing committees for such organizations as the American Heart Association and Cancer Society, and they act as preceptors or mentors for both undergraduate and graduate nursing students.

## History

As nursing service moved from centralization to decentralization, it became clear that more staff development would be necessary. Two important needs were identified:

1. The increasing responsibility being assumed by staff nurses and head nurses meant that certain nursing skills required additional development. Nurses needed to expand their body of knowledge in order to make independent high-quality patient-care decisions and to interact within our decentralized environment.
2. The growing independence and increased authority and responsibility assumed by head nurses meant that leadership skills were a paramount necessity. Head nurses and assistant head nurses needed more management training.

As a result of this latter requirement, a Management and Organizational Development (MOD) program was initiated.

## MOD

Known at El Camino as MOD, our management and organizational development program is intended to improve the management skills of all nurses, but it is directed particularly toward head nurses. A two-year program, it requires attendance at two-day workshops away from the hospital once every three months. Participants include head nurses, assistant head nurses, nursing coordinators, and staff development instructors, as well as all managers and supervisors from other hospital departments.

A new series of MOD groups starts twice a year to provide training in management theory and skills for employees who are moving into leadership positions. This allows new managers to take part in, and have access to, the same management theory as do their peers.

Workshops are informal, with a minimum of lectures. They use a fully participative experiential learning model. Real data from the workplace is incorporated into the program as often as possible, and there are specific assignments for practicing new skills on the job.

Both first-line supervision (assistant head nurse) and middle management (head-nurse) topics are covered. Some examples include the following:

- Leadership—the awareness of one's own style, motivation, and so on.
- Communication—interpersonal, group, and in meetings.
- Job clarification—coaching, performance review.
- Time management.
- Personnel aspects of supervision—including hiring and firing
- Creative problem solving and decision making.
- Management cycle goals and objective setting.

An outside consultant was hired to develop the MOD program. He worked very closely with staff development instructors, who functioned as cotrainers and coordinators of the program within the hospital. MOD now continues under the direction of a full-time management and organizational development trainer employed by El Camino Hospital.

Following the commitment to participative management, a design committee for MOD was established. This committee consists of a permanent core group made up of the director of education and training, the MOD trainer, the director of personnel, and the director of management engineering. Also included are representatives who serve on a rotating basis from different areas of the hospital. The purpose of the committee is to recommend the content, format, and time frames of the MOD sessions to hospital administration. For example, one of the committee's recommendations was that all department heads become proficient in leading meetings. As administration agreed with this assessment, one of the first programs presented in MOD was on conducting effective meetings.

MOD has been instrumental in changing the way our organization works because it provides a common management theory, philosophy, and language. Since much of our organization's work is accomplished in meetings, the program on leading meetings has had a dramatic impact. Meeting participants are notified of the purpose of each meeting. Leaders do preparatory work, describe the purpose of the meeting again to participants, explain what their roles will be, establish the ground rules, and make clear assignments to participants. At the end of each meeting, participants are asked to evaluate the proceedings. Use of chart pads for brainstorming or recording discussions allows all to see progress of the meeting and facilitates ease in recording minutes. Seldom now do we hear such comments as, "That meeting was a waste of my time!"

In addition to the eight basic workshops of the MOD program, six other training events are offered each year to allow managers to keep abreast of new ideas and skills. These have included a rapid-reading course, an update in coaching skills, and a seminar on writing effectiveness.

With decentralization accelerating at El Camino, MOD remains an important tool in staff development. It not only allows for an increase in skills and knowledge, but also provides a valuable vehicle for problem solving and team building.

## CLINICALLY ORIENTED STAFF DEVELOPMENT

Increasing staff-nurse skill with patient care was the other major need identified during the transition to decentralization. This is being provided through the following means:

- Staff Development Instructor support in each complex on all three shifts.
- Clinical skill validation.
- Independent self-paced learning (learning center).

Patient care decisions are made and updated on each shift. Therefore the availability of educational resources to practitioners on all three shifts is an important component in the effectiveness of decentralization. Educational support in the form of instructors varies, however, according to complex size and numbers of instructors assigned to each complex (see Exhibit 6-2).

Medical-Surgical-Orthopedics, the largest nursing complex, has instructors assigned to each shift. In the other complexes instructors have responsibility for educational coverage on all three shifts. These instructors work an "overlap" shift once a week. This is a combination evening/night shift, which provides support to nurses working those shifts.

Time spent on the clinical unit is a high priority for staff development in providing educational support to the staff. Each instructor spends a designated amount of time every week on each clinical unit for which she or he has educational responsibility. This varies from one to four hours per week. While the instructors do often assist with patient care during their clinical unit time, they do not take a patient assignment. Their primary role is education— not helping the unit to meet its staffing needs. The clinical unit time is spent in a variety of ways, with the emphasis given to validation of nursing skills for staff. For instance, an instructor may spend this time:

1. demonstrating (or validating for a staff nurse) a complete physical exam of a patient's chest,

**Exhibit 6-2.  Staff Development Instructors
Assigned Units and Shifts**

| | | |
|---|---|---|
| Maternal-Child Instructor | Labor & Delivery<br>Post-Partum<br>Nursery | all<br>three<br>shifts |
| Dialysis Instructor | Artificial Kidney Unit<br>Home Training Unit<br>Continuous Ambulatory<br>Peritoneal Dialysis<br>Resource to 5 West (for inpatient<br>kidney) | two shifts<br>day shift<br>day shift<br><br>all shifts |
| Critical Care Instructor | Intensive Care Unit<br>Transitional Care Unit | all three<br>shifts |
| Critical Care Instructor | Emergency Room<br>Coronary Care Unit | all three<br>shifts |
| Medical-Surgical-<br>Orthopedic Instructor | 2 Surgical Units<br>1 Surgical-Short Term<br>1 Orthopedics Unit<br>1 Kidney/GU Unit | day<br>shift |
| Medical-Surgical-<br>Orthopedic Instructor | 2 Medical Units<br>1 Surgical/GYN Unit<br>1 Pediatrics Unit | day<br>shift |
| Medical-Surgical-<br>Orthopedic-Instructor | 2 Surgical Units<br>1 Surgical-Short Term<br>1 Surgical/GYN Unit<br>1 Kidney/GU Unit | evenings |
| Medical-Surgical-<br>Orthopedic Instructor | 1 Orthopedics Unit<br>2 Medical Units<br>1 Pediatrics Unit | nights |

2. validating an analysis of EKG rhythm strips,
3. certifying a hyperalimentation resource nurse,
4. assisting with formulation of a patient care plan,
5. reviewing equipment on the crash cart,
6. helping log roll a patient,
7. discussing implications of lab results on a kidney dialysis patient,
8. trouble-shooting an overly sensitive infusion pump,

9. demonstrating patient teaching with a baby bath,
10. coaching a preceptor and a new employee, and
11. meeting with staff to revise the unit's core curriculum.

Theoretical knowledge is provided by instructors through classroom instruction, seminars, and workshops. However, this method of program development and teaching is very time consuming and takes the instructor away from the clincal unit. The creation of educational modules, utilizing the concepts of self-paced learning, is advantageous to both instructors and staff.

## EDUCATIONAL MODULES

An educational module is a complete, independent, educational program. Modules support El Camino's belief that learning is a lifelong process and that each nurse is responsible for his or her own learning. Adult learning principles, including the idea that the best learning takes place if accomplished at the time of need, are incorporated into the modules.

Modules include a list of objectives, a pre-test, the content area, a post-test, and an evaluation. A variety of audiovisual media may be used to expand the written portion of the modules. A module may be totally printed in form, or it may be in combination with an audiotape, slides, videocassette, or filmstrip. Modules at El Camino also contain a "patient care component" whenever relevent. This requires that a nurse perform a return skill demonstration with or for a patient and have this skill validated by a staff development instructor or resoruce nurse. For instance, a nurse may go through the six-part chest-exam module, after which she or he must do a complete physical exam of the chest on at least one patient, and have a staff development instructor validate this skill.

In terms of both the nurse/learner's needs and the staff development instructor's time, independent self-paced learning appears to be the most effective and efficient teaching/learning method. Modules do not require the assistance of an instructor. This convenience allows nurses to go through modules whenever they like. Because a module is immediately available, the nurse has access to its content when she or he has the learning need—no need to wait six weeks while the instructor develops and teaches a program. If the module contains new or difficult material, the nurse may repeat the module several times, until she or he feels comfortable that the material has been mastered. This is difficult, if not impossible, to do in a classroom setting. Modules are also advantageous to the instructors, relieving them of repetitious teaching and allowing them more time for clinical unit validating skills or the development of new educational programs in the module format.

Modules have been developed for new employees going through orientation and for experienced nurses who need ready access to new content.

Modules developed for orientation include such titles as "IV Therapy," "Fluid and Electrolytes," "The California Nurse Practice Act," and "Care Planning." Some of the modules developed for the experienced nurse are "Care of the Patient on Hyperalimentation," "Care of the Patient with Vascular Access Device," and a series called "Physical Assessment of the Adult."

These modules may also be completed for continuing education credit, a benefit that assists the nursing staff in meeting the California mandatory continuing education requirement for relicensure.

### LEARNING CENTER

To support the concept of independent, self-paced learning, El Camino hospital has established a learning center under the auspices of staff development. Representatives from all levels of nursing service were asked to participate in the planning committee that coordinated the development of the center—a project which took a year to complete. Thus staff were involved in both planning and the implementation of the learning center as an in-house educational tool.

The center is a quiet, attractive, comfortable room equipped with video-cassettes, filmstrips, and slide-sound programs. Not all programs are formalized into modules, but many have accompanying written materials or study guides. Programs and equipment are adapted for use by individuals or for small groups of up to four persons. The master list of programs lists each program stored in the learning center, indicating the title and the type of medium through which the program is available.

Upon employment, each nurse receives an introduction to the learning center as part of his or her hospital orientation. This is a valuable resource for the new employee—one that will be used immediately, because many parts of the orientation are in modules housed in the center. In addition to the formal orientation, printed instructions are available to assist the nurse in use of the equipment. If this information is not sufficient, the nurse may request assistance from a member of staff development. There is no librarian or technician to staff the learning center. To provide easy staff access to the learning center plus security for equipment and materials stored there, a combination lock is used. All staff have access to the combination numbers for the lock. Thus nurses may use the learning center any time, day or night, seven days a week. Nurses may go through programs at times convenient to them, each at an appropriate, individual pace.

The learning center was developed to improve and maintain nursing skills for high-quality patient care. We have been very pleased with its success in this regard. Nurses also utilize the learning center for their own growth and development. For instance, nurses complete programs in the learning center to change thier nursing specialties.

The learning center may be used by staff on their own time. Use on paid time, however, is often the result of an agreement or contract between a staff nurse and head nurse—to meet an identified learning need.

All staff have input into the selection of the materials placed in the learning center. Staff development instructors, however, take the responsibility for providing the rationale that justifies the cost of the programs and materials selected. This rationale is usually based on identfied learning needs.

## LEARNING NEEDS ASSESSMENT

Learning needs of staff are identified in a variety of ways. While nurses themselves are expected to identify their own learning needs, staff development instructors are expected to provide the mechanisms or tools needed for accomplishing a learning needs assessment.

A needs assessment may be done informally and verbally, or formally through written questionnaires or quality assurance data. A staff nurse may say, "I need X skill to be a competent nurse on this unit." A head nurse may note "Forty percent of our patients are over 65 years of age, and my staff is not well-grounded in gerontological nursing principles." A staff nurse who transfers to another unit may see a need and suggest that nurses learn a new skill. Staff development instructors may attend a conference or workshop that indicates a new standard of practice is evolving. Quality assurance coordinators may detect needs through patient-care incident reports and nursing-care audits. If the deficiencies detected through the nursing audit are determined to be a knowledge or skill problem, then the head nurse may ask staff development to assist in developing a remedial plan of action.

For example, there may have been an increase in the number of IV-medication errors on a nursing unit. This could be a problem resulting from several different causes: not enough staff, nurses not checking for the correct patient, physicians ordering new or unfamiliar medications, physicians writing confusing orders, or one of several other possibilities. Suppose, after collecting data, the head nurse finds the problem is lack of knowledge about IV medications given at this hospital. She or he decides to ask the unit's staff development instructor to prepare an appropriate educational program to remedy the problem. After the educational program is implemented, quality assurance is asked to do an audit to determine if the program was effective and if the needs assessment was appropriate.

Staff development instructors often are able to identify informally the learning needs of staff during their scheduled weekly clinical unit time. Also, periodically—usually at least once a year—instructors ask the staff to fill out an individual needs assessment questionnaire. This data is given to the head nurse, and used by the head nurse and staff development instructor in planning and contracting for educational programs and support for the unit.

Besides personal observation and data collection, two tools are routinely used to assist the staff and head nurses in identifying real or potential learning needs. One is the *skills inventory,* which is initally filled out by all nurses during their orientation period; the other is the *core curriculum.*

## Skills Inventory

The skills inventory is a checklist of nursing skills, both technical and process, which have been found to be necessary for nurses to function adequately on any given nursing unit. Separate inventories have been developed for each of the complexes in the hospital. In addition, there are addendums for specific nursing units with special skill requirements—i.e., traction for the orthopedic unit is attached to the general MSO skills inventory. A *master skills inventory* is a further refinement of the skills inventory. With emphasis on staff input, each head nurse develops a master skills inventory for the unit. Using the skills inventory for the complex, she or he determines which skills are absolutely essential for the specific unit. These skills are indicated on the skills inventory by an asterisk.

Each skills inventory has the same basic design. The form (see Exhibit 6–3) is divided into three columns. The first is headed "Self Assessment." Here nurses rank themselves by answering such questions as, "Have I ever done this procedure before?" "Do I feel competent in doing this procedure?" "Could I teach someone else this procedure?"

Column two is headed "El Camino Hospital Protocol." This is to be checked off after the nurses have first looked up the appropriate procedure in the procedure Rolodex and discussed it with their preceptor. (A preceptor is a staff nurse who provides the majority of support given to the new employee during clinical unit orientation. For a more detailed explanation, see the section entitled "Preceptors" later in this chapter.) Since each hospital has its own style of accomplishing the same procedure, this assessment is to determine if the nurses' previous experience matches the protocol at El Camino. If not, do they understand why and how to do it here?

The third column is "Validated by Preceptor." This indicates that the preceptor has supervised the new employee the first time she or he accomplished the procedure at El Camino. The preceptor must validate all skills on the master skills inventory for the unit, since these have been identified by the head nurse as essential to safe patient care on that unit. The preceptor may also elect to validate any other skill on the inventory as a means of evaluating the progress of the new employee's orientation.

Ideally, the skills inventory should be completed during the orientation period; it *must* be completed before the end of the probationary period. The skills inventory is kept in the employee's file on the nursing unit for periodic updating. Thus the individual nurse is responsible for seeing that all required skills are learned and validated. The skills inventory also may be used as a tool for evaluating a new employee at the end of the three-month probationary employment period.

## Core Curriculum

Another resource utilized for assessing learning needs of new employees is the core curriculum. Core curriculum is a collection of individualized self-paced educational activities kept on the nursing unit. Nurses are expected to carry out these activities with the assistance of their preceptors, head nurses, and staff development instructors. Each subject area has written objectives to be accomplished by the nurse, followed by activities that will assist the nurse in meeting the objectives. These activities may be as simple as reading a journal article or as complex as going through a series of modules on a given subject. A variety of resources are utilized: the learning center; books, journals, and manuals; and instruction at the bedside. The following is taken from the core curriculum for Medical-Surgical-Orthopedics:

> Essentially, the Core Curriculum (Level I) is a set of *basic* theoretically oriented learning experiences which encompass nursing process and technical skills which must be successfully completed by all RNs at El Camino Hospital to insure professional quality patient care.
>
> The curriculum is progressive, beginning in general hospital orientation, and continuing through the nurses' probationary period. In the event expectations have not been met at the end of that period, objectives are written which include timeframes and outcomes.

Priorities and expectations for the curriculum are determined by head nurses with input from staff development instructors in accordance with unit/complex needs and goals.

The following is an example of one objective of the curriculum, developed specifically for the Gyn unit:

### Suprapubic Catheter

*Objectives*

1. Verbalizes rationale for the need for S.P. catheter.
2. Demonstrates appropriate techniques (as described in S.P. catheter program) for S.P. catheter routine and care.
3. Describes available resources for the care of the patient with an S.P. catheter.

**Exhibit 6-3.    Partial Skills Inventory**

| | SELF ASSESS-MENT | ECH PROTO-COL | VALIDATED BY PRECEPTOR | REMARKS |
|---|---|---|---|---|
| I. ASSISTANCE WITH PROCEDURES | | | | |
| A. Sigmoidoscopy | | | | |
| B. Pelvic examination | | | | |
| C. Chest tube insertion and removal | | | | |
| D. Dressing change | | | | |
| E. Paracentesis | | | | |
| F. Thorancentesis | | | | |
| G. Joint aspirations | | | | |
| H. Lumbar puncture | | | | |
| I. CVP insertion and removal | | | | |
| J. Cutdowns | | | | |
| K. Physical examination | | | | |
| L. Bone-marrow biopsy | | | | |
| M. Liver biopsy | | | | |
| N. Phlebotomy | | | | |
| O. Endotracheal intubation | | | | |
| II. EXPERIENCE IN USING EQUIPMENT (Purpose, maintenance, trouble shooting) | | | | |
| A. Hypothermia blanket | | | | |
| B. Alternating pressure mattress | | | | |
| C. Restraints | | | | |
| D. Bed board | | | | |
| E. Foot board | | | | |
| F. Cradles | | | | |
| G. Guerneys (new x-ray guerney) | | | | |
| H. Electric beds | | | | |

**Exhibit 6-3.** *(continued)*

| | SELF ASSESS-MENT | ECH PROTO-COL | VALIDATED BY PRECEPTOR | REMARKS |
|---|---|---|---|---|
| I. Straight suction | | | | |
| J. Foley care | | | | |
|    1. Foley insertion | | | | |
|    2. Foley removal | | | | |
|    3. Foley irrigation | | | | |
| K. Suprapubic catheter care (2N) | | | | |
|    1. Clamping procedure | | | | |
|    2. Irrigation procedure | | | | |
|    3. Dressings | | | | |
| L. Skin suture removal | | | | |
| M. Decubitus care | | | | |
| N. Stump care | | | | |
| O. Crutch walking (5E) (5W) | | | | |
| P. Cast care | | | | |
| Q. Post-mortem care | | | | |
| R. Seizure precautions | | | | |
| S. Personal hygiene | | | | |
| T. Chest tube (6E, 6W, 2E, 2W, 3W) | | | | |
|    1. Drainage system | | | | |
|      a. Pleurevac | | | | |
|      b. Emerson | | | | |
|    2. Trouble shooting | | | | |
| U. Special feeding techniques | | | | |
|    1. Rubber-tipped syringe | | | | |
|    2. Gastrostomy | | | | |
|    3. N/G tube | | | | |
|    4. Feeding patient with a tracheostomy | | | | |

*Note:* The list presented here is not a comprehensive skills inventory.

*Learning Activities*
  1. Will view and complete three-part program (slide/sound module) on suprapubic catheters in the Learning Center, SL 219.
  2. Will be able to return demonstrate for preceptor the techniques and criteria listed in the suprapubic catheter program.

The curriculum was developed and is updated by staff development instructors with assistance from head nurses and staff nurses. At present, only Level I (basic) of the curriculum has been developed. It is anticipated, however, that Level II (advanced) will be developed in the future to assist nurses in acquiring more advanced skills.


## ORIENTATION

El Camino's philosophy regarding orientation states the following:
"The orientation period for the new employee is critical. Development as a competent professional is a result of the basic introduction received during orientation. The new employee must become fully knowledgeable of the specific policies, procedures, and patient population in order to give specialized patient care."

El Camino's philosophy incorporates the belief that a thorough, supportive orientation is a necessity. In a supportive atmosphere new employees learn that their coworkers (and the institution) care about patients, and care about them and their success as employees. Realizing that a comprehensive orientation is directly related to retention of new staff, El Camino Hospital has made a large commitment in time, energy, and money toward the orientation of new employees.

Staff development is responsible for the orientation of new employees and for the incorporation of hospital philosophy into the orientation process. A new employee hired into the nursing service at El Camino is given a structured orientation, which is then individualized at the unit level. Upon employment, the head nurse determines how much orientation the new employee will need by utilizing established guidelines. She or he takes into account the new nurse's experience, education, and previous employment. For an experienced RN, orientation is usually three weeks. The majority of new nurses hired at El Camino begin their employment on the evening or night shifts. Their orientation, however, begins on the day shift. Day-shift orientation includes general hospital orientation, general nursing orientation, and the initial nursing-unit orientation. This covers a two-week period.

The third week of a new employee's orientation is then spent on the shift for which she or he has been hired. The exception to this rule is the new graduate nurse. New graduates spend the first two months of a three-month orientation on days.

The first day of orientation is spent in getting acquainted with the hospital. New nurses are oriented with all new hospital employees to electrical safety, disaster drill requirements, time cards, and employee benefits. The next three days are spent in general nursing orientation, which includes a visit to and discussion of the learning center. New nurses are introduced to the MIS (medical information system) computer, and certified in basic CPR (Cardio-pulmonary Resuscitation) and in IV Therapy. They are familiarized with the philosophy of decentralized nursing, the California Nurse Practice Act, and the preceptor program at El Camino. The next several days are utilized in orientation to the nursing unit and patient care. During the third week of orientation, another full day is spent in general nursing orientation. This includes care planning, quality assurance and audit, charting policies, infor-mation on infection control, and, finally, an evaluation of the orientation experience.

The remainder of the orientation period is spent on the clinical nursing unit. The new employee is not counted as staff while being oriented and thus is not responsible for a patient assignment or counted in the patient acuities. While not responsible for a patient assignment, she or he will give care as a means of learning procedures, becoming familiar with equipment, developing organizational skills, and learning the hospital's philosophy of patient care, as shown in Exhibit 6-4.

An important component in the clinical unit orientation of a new employee is the preceptor program.

**Preceptors**

A preceptor is a staff nurse who provides the majority of support given to the new employee during his/her clinical unit orientation. The preceptor is a "buddy"—and much, much more. As another staff nurse, the preceptor is a peer who has the responsibility of teaching and guiding the new employee's experiences, of providing ongoing feedback about progress, and, finally, of assisting the head nurse and assistant head nurse with the new employee's initial formal evaluation.

To accomplish the training which they must provide for new employees, preceptors are given a certain amount of training hours or release time (from patient care) by the head nurse. Over a three-week orientation period, the preceptor may have as many as 30 hours of time to work with the new nurse. Experience has shown that the new nurse needs more of the preceptor's time during the first few days of employment. For example, four hours are usually spent during the first day the preceptor and new nurse are together on the clinical unit. Thereafter they may spend two hours a day for several days. Toward the end of orientation, this may drop to only one hour per day. Initially the preceptor and new employee take two or three patients to care for

**Exhibit 6–4.    El Camino Hospital Nursing Service Orientation**

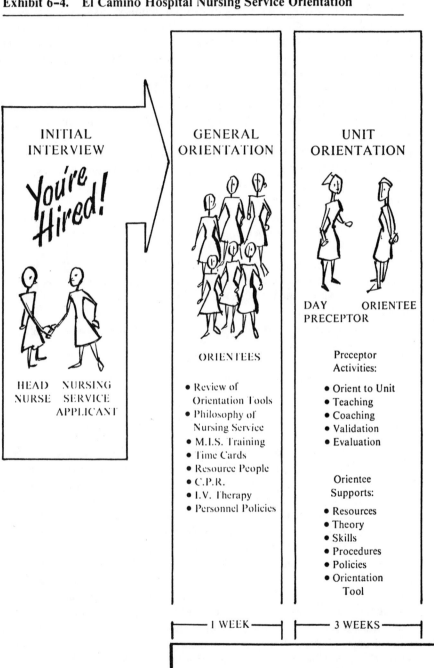

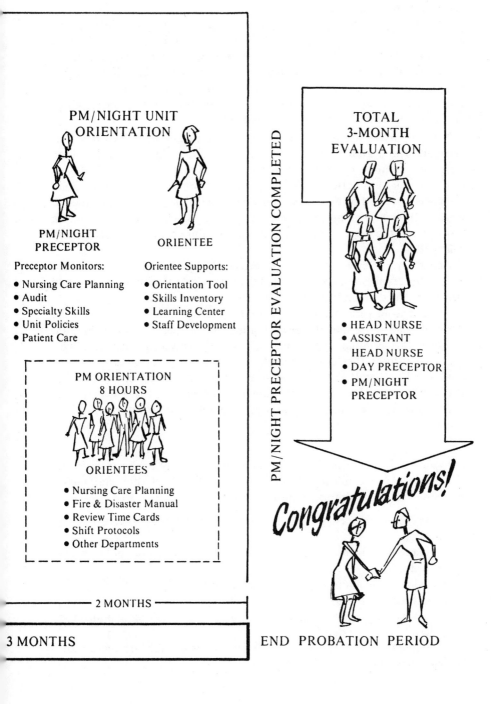

PM/NIGHT UNIT ORIENTATION

PM/NIGHT PRECEPTOR

ORIENTEE

Preceptor Monitors:
• Nursing Care Planning
• Audit
• Specialty Skills
• Unit Policies
• Patient Care

Orientee Supports:
• Orientation Tool
• Skills Inventory
• Learning Center
• Staff Development

PM ORIENTATION 8 HOURS

ORIENTEES
• Nursing Care Planning
• Fire & Disaster Manual
• Review Time Cards
• Shift Protocols
• Other Departments

PM/NIGHT PRECEPTOR EVALUATION COMPLETED

TOTAL 3-MONTH EVALUATION

• HEAD NURSE
• ASSISTANT HEAD NURSE
• DAY PRECEPTOR
• PM/NIGHT PRECEPTOR

Congratulations!

2 MONTHS

3 MONTHS

END PROBATION PERIOD

together. By the end of orientation, new nurses will be working independently. They should be ready to assume a full patient load and will now be counted in the patient acuities.

The time that a preceptor uses for training is calculated as part of the acuities for a unit. For example, if the preceptor plans to spend four hours a day with a new nurse for the first two days of clinical employment, the preceptor will be counted as .5 (or one-half person) for two days. If the normal patient load for that person is four to six patients (depending on the patients' acuity), then during the days of preceptorship, the preceptor will be responsible for a patient load of two or three patients.

New employees will have one preceptor with them during their day-shift orientation and another preceptor on the shift to which they have been assigned—evenings or nights. Before leaving the day shift, new employees receive formal evaluation from their day-shift preceptors. The evaluation usually is discussed by the day-shift preceptor with the preceptor assigned to work with the new employee on evenings or nights. This provides a smooth transition to the permanent shift and prevents duplication of skills already validated.

Under certain circumstances the orientation period may be extended beyond the usual established period of time. This is done with reluctance, and only when the data indicates the nurse has great potential.

At the end of three weeks of orientation, the preceptor meets with the assistant head nurse and the new employee for a final formal evaluation. Although this terminates the formal relationship between the new employee and the preceptor, they usually maintain close ties. The new nurse is encouraged to ask any staff nurse for assistance, not only during orientation but afterward as well. Experience has shown, however, that the new employee generally turns to the preceptor as a primary resource for information and guidance.

*Preceptor Selection and Training.* As preceptors play a vital role in the orientation of new employees, head nurses select them with care. Staff nurses are chosen to be preceptors because they are

1. expert practitioners, possessing good technical and process nursing skills;
2. permanent full-time employees, familiar with hospital policies and procedures;
3. knowledgeable about appropriate resources;
4. good teachers, or have a desire to teach;
5. nurses who enjoy working in a close, one-to-one teaching relationship;
6. eager to accept responsibility;
7. prepared to be a preceptor, having attended the one-day preceptor training workshop.

To prepare nurses to be preceptors after they have been selected by their head nurse, staff development provides a one-day workshop. The workshop is scheduled two or three times a year, depending on the need for the new preceptors. Nurses are required to attend the workshop (at hospital expense) before they precept. As an added benefit, a nurse may take the workshop for continuing-education credit.

The content in the workshop includes an overview of orientation, the use of learning-needs-assessment and evaluation tools, the roles and responsibilities of the new employee and preceptor, and the functions of the head nurse, the assistant head nurse, and the staff development instructor (see Exhibit 6–5). Also included in the workshop are principles of adult learning, assessment of the learner, writing of behavioral objectives, how to give feedback, and the use of evaluation techniques.

Role-playing exercises are utilized in the workshop to assist the new preceptors in developing skill in giving negative feedback—one of the most difficult areas in precepting.

After completion of the workshop, the preceptor is assigned to the next new nurse employed on the unit. During his or her first experience, the new preceptor has a preceptor—a staff development instructor. Giving support to the preceptors and new employees has high priority, and staff development instructors are available to assist the preceptor at any time. This help may take the form of assistance in writing behavioral objectives, in problem solving, in coaching, or in validating preceptor techniques. It is important that preceptors receive feedback that tells them what they are doing is valid and appropriate for the new employee.

The head nurse and assistant head nurse also provide support to the preceptor. Assurance of training time and monitoring of the new employee's progress are provided. Suggestions and well-deserved praise are given to the preceptor.

As with all employees, the new nurse is expected to be self-directed, to act as an adult learner, and to take responsibility for his or her own learning. New nurses are expected to give their preceptors feedback about what they need to learn, and whether the pace is appropriate. Of course preceptors are expected to play an active role in assisting new employees in identifying their learning needs; preceptors are familiar with the physicians, with unit routines, and with the usual types of patients. Again, to facilitate the process of identifying learning needs, the skills inventory and the core curriculum are utilized.

Following orientation, new employees are asked to evaluate the performance of their preceptor. As this is a growth experience for the preceptor, she or he is eager for feedback. The staff development instructor also provides feedback to the preceptor regarding his or her effectiveness in the new role.

At El Camino Hospital, preceptors are included in the group of experts called "resource nurses."

**Exhibit 6-5.   Orientation Responsibilities Guidelines**

| | HEAD NURSE | PRECEPTOR | NURSE EDUCATOR | NEW EMPLOYEE |
|---|---|---|---|---|
| ASSESSMENT | 1. Interviews and hires new employees with input from AHN<br>2. Administers Clinical Unit Skills Inventory<br>3. Pre-tests for theory and clinical abilities<br>4. Compares new employee to competencies in CORE Curriculum | 1. Reviews results of and explains use of:<br>• Clinical Skills Inventory<br>• CORE Curriculum<br>• Objectives<br>• Other tests given with new employees<br>2. Direct observation of new employee clinical performance | 1. Reviews results of<br>• Clinical Skills Inventory<br>• CORE Curriculum<br>• Other tests given<br>2. Direct observation of new employee performance | 1. Completes and updates Clinical Skills Inventory self assessment of current performance level<br>2. Identifies own learning needs |
| PLANNING | 1. Selects preceptor for new employee<br>2. Informs nursing education, preceptor & unit staff of new employee's hire date and learning needs<br>3. Assigns new employee to orient day shift and/or off shift | 1. Has planning conference with new employee first clinical day<br>2. Writes mutually agreed upon goals and objectives to increase skill and performance level of new employee | 1. Informs preceptor & unit of first clinical day<br>2. Assists preceptor in writing goals & objectives | 1. Writes mutually agreed upon goals and objectives with preceptor |

| | | | | |
|---|---|---|---|---|
| **IMPLEMENTATION** | 1. Provides orientation and preceptor time for new employee | 1. Is not "in charge" while precepting<br>2. Provides learning-center time for new employee<br>3. Provides learning activities for new employees<br>4. Acts as clinical resource for new employee<br>5. Weekly conferences to review progress on technical and process skills<br>6. Gives ongoing feedback regarding performance<br>7. Validates skills according to protocol | 1. Provides new employee with general hospital orientation<br>2. Provides preceptors with preceptor training program<br>3. Assists preceptor in locating appropriate learning activities | 1. Reads procedure & policy manuals<br>2. Initiates own learning experiences<br>3. Follows learning activities outlined in CORE Curriculum and follows "Guidelines for Integrating Nursing Process into Practice" |
| **EVALUATION** | 1. Evaluates orientee's progress by observation & feedback from orientee and preceptor<br>2. Conducts 3-month evaluation conference with preceptor and new employee<br>3. Determines if orientation needs to be extended<br>4. Assigns new employee to permanent status | 1. Conferences with new employees about progress at end of orientation<br>2. Gives feedback to RN regarding new employees' performance<br>3. Provides written evaluation to new employee using<br>goals & objectives<br>direct observation<br>clinical unit skills inventory<br>Process-to-Practice tool | 1. Assists preceptor & new employee in evaluating new employee's progress<br>2. Consults on any proposed extension of probation or orientation<br>3. Evaluates orientation and updates learning programs as needed<br>4. Reviews orientation evaluations and gives feedback to preceptors and head nurses | 1. Conferences with head nurse and preceptor at end or orientation<br>2. Evaluates preceptor program and orientation<br>3. Writes self evaluation of progress with use of Clinical Unit Skills Inventory, & mutually set goals & objectives |

## Resource Nurses

The development of the resource-nurse concept was an extension of the philosophy of decentralization, which calls for more decision making at the staff-nurse level. A resource nurse is a nurse who is an experienced practitioner and has specialized knowledge pertinent to a diagnosis or particular group of patients. In a decentralized structure, each nurse shares expertise with colleagues, and every patient has the right to expect optimal care from his or her nurse. Reality, however, is that every nurse cannot be all things to all patients. To bridge this gap, the concept of the resource nurse evolved. These nurses act as resources for other nurses, for patients, and for patients' families.

There are resource nurses in all nursing complexes. For instance, a diabetic resource nurse may work on Pediatrics, Surgical, Medical, Intensive Care, or Gynecology. In fact, the first group to evolve was the diabetic resource nurses, whose primary goal is to improve the care of the diabetic patient. These nurses assess diabetic patients, make patient-care recommendations to the patient and his/her family, suggest hospital and community resources, assist in family and patient teaching, and help with discharge planning.

In addition, there are now resource nurse groups for arterial blood gases (ABG), hyperalimentation, ostomies, and vascular access devices (cannula care). In each of these areas, certification of skills is required, with revalidation of skills each year.

The certification process includes attendance at a required educational program, which may take the form of a workshop or may be designated programs in the learning center. This is then followed by a skill demonstration or return demonstration on a patient or group of patients. For instance, to become a certified hyperalimentation resource nurse, a nurse must take a pre-test, read a written module on special-care needs of a patient on hyperalimentation, view a slide/sound program on protocol for dressing and tubing changes, complete two dressing and tubing changes under the supervision of a staff development instructor, and pass a written post-test. Successful completion of this criteria gives the nurse certification as a hyperalimentation resource nurse.

To meet an identified need, resource nurse support groups were formed. These groups meet periodically for the purpose of keeping members up to date on the latest information and techniques and to provide emotional support for one another.

The head nurse often contracts with a staff nurse on the unit for that nurse to become a resource nurse; then the staff nurse and head nurse both contract with their staff development instructor to accomplish this activity.

*Contracting.* Staff Development Instructors utilize contracts to establish a formal agreement on how a learning need will be met. Such a learning contract is usually developed between a head nurse and a staff development instructor, but it may also be with an assistant head nurse or staff nurse or group of staff nurses. A contract may also exist between the director of nursing service and staff development, when the learning need or goal involves more than one nursing complex—for instance, certifying all nursing service personnel in CPR.

Long-term goals and objectives are first determined by the organization, and then followed by a contract between the director of nursing service and each of the head nurses. The head nurse then negotiates with the staff development instructor for educational activities needed to meet these goals and objectives.

While each contract varies in who accepts responsibility for each of the components, certain responsibilities are automatically assumed by either the head nurse or the instructor.

The staff development instructor assists in the learning needs assessment, determines the best educational methods to use, develops an educational program, implements the program, and assists in the evaluation of the program and its cost effectiveness.

The head nurse is responsible for assisting in the learning needs assessment, determining how high a priority the learning need is, and ensuring that the new skill will be used with patients on the unit. She or he also assists in program evaluation.

Negotiations are important in each of these aspects, and may also include such factors as a determination of how much instruction time is needed—both initially and for the follow-up coaching and validation of the skill on the unit—and the determiniation of who will validate the newly learned skill.

Another factor is the determiniation of who needs to learn the skill—two resource nurses on each shift, for example, or all full-time staff. Do *all* staff need to learn the skill? If all staff must learn the skill, usually the head nurse, assistant head nurses, and preceptors go through the program first. Then they act as resources and role models for the rest of the staff.

One program that was developed as a result of this process is the physical assessment of the chest. Several head nurses identified the need for their staff to be able to perform a chest assessment on a patient with respiratory disease and report their findings. This need arose as a result of an increase in the number of respiratory patients being cared for on those units. Staff development instructors developed a six-part module, "Chest Assessment." Initially the program was taught in a six-hour workshop for head nurses, and assistant head nurses. The program was then placed in the learning center. Each staff nurse on those units contracted with the staff development instructor to complete the program. After completion of the module, skills were practiced and validated by staff development instructors.

Contracts may also be of a more general nature, to provide educational support for ongoing objectives—i.e., maintenance of care planning, discharge teaching, and so on. These contracts are for six months to one year, and are reviewed and renewed.

As noted earlier, cardiopulmonary resuscitation (CPR) is one contract that staff development maintains with the director of nursing services—to provide certification and recertification of this skill for all employees within nursing service.

*CPR.* A three-hour course in CPR, using American Heart Association standards, is provided as part of the general nursing orientation. Also included in the training are things specific to El Camino Hospital, such as the emergency telephone number, a discussion of the roles and responsibilities of each member of the CPR team, and a review of the crash cart. Each orientee must successfully return demonstrate one- and two-man adult resuscitation techniques, as well as resuscitation of the infant.

All nursing personnel are expected to be recertified yearly in basic CPR. To accomplish this, staff development offers a CPR "marathon" four times a year. It is called a marathon because classes are offered on the hour, every hour, on all three shifts, for two days. The staff see a video tape on CPR, and then must successfully return demonstrate one- and two-man rescue of the adult and resuscitate the infant, then pass a test on finding equipment on the crash cart within a certain time frame. After successful completion, a colored dot is placed next to the person's name on the staffing board in the staffing office. Thus head nurses (and all) can see quickly who has been recertified in CPR in any given year—and who needs to be recertified.

El Camino Hospital is a community hospital without 24-hour physician coverage, so a CPR team concept is utilized. The team functions in lieu of physician, if one is not immediately available, providing emergency care to a patient who has suffered a cardiac arrest. CPR protocols and standing orders have been developed that allow nurses to provide patients with emergency care until a physician arrives. The team is led by an experienced CCU nurse. Responsibilities for administering medications, providing massage, and recording CPR events are shared and rotated through the MSO nursing units. Respiratory therapists ventilate the patient in a Code CPR when an anesthesiologist is not available; at least one therapist per shift must be certified to perform intubations. The CPR team is utilized on all three shifts and responds to all paged code CPRs. When a physician responds, he assumes responsibility for leading the Code, and the CCU nurse becomes a resource for both the physician and the rest of the CPR team.

In orientation, nurses receive the basic CPR training that enables them to initiate resuscitation efforts on their patients. Nurses are not expected to be CPR team members, however, until they have completed at least the probationary period (three months). At that time, MSO nurses attend a two-hour class to prepare them to participate as a CPR team member. The class includes information on how to set priorities in a Code, how to administer medications—what and how much are protocol medications, and responsibilities of the massage nurse and the recorder. They also view a video tape of mock Code CPR.

Mock Code CPR drills are set up monthly, rotating from unit to unit. These drills give both unit personnel and CPR team members experience in responding to codes. Mock codes are paged over the PA system as "mock Code CPRs" with personnel responding to them just as if they were the real thing. These drills are particularly helpful to new or inexperienced staff. Staff development instructors initiate the mock codes and assist in the critiques afterwards. Instructors also respond to all paged actual emergencies, acting as a resource to staff and assisting in any way needed.

Staff development also offers courses in advanced cardiac life support (ACLS). These courses are offered several times each year to provide critical-care nurses and physicians with required certification.

*Health Education.* Another group of nurses in the hospital provides consultation services to patients and staff. These consultation services are in the areas of patient teaching and preventative medicine and are available through the health education department.

Health education is a division within the department of education and training. The name—health education—was chosen to reinforce the preventative medicine concept. The emphasis for the department is divided into three areas: patient education, community/industrial education, and health enhancement classes for hospital staff.

Health education supports the philosophy of decentralization in nursing by providing consultation services to the practitioner at the bedside—particularly in the area of patient teaching. An example might be a patient who is hospitalized with severe back pain. The responsible nurse assesses the patient, including learning needs. If she or he believes this patient may need more intensive teaching than time permits, the responsible nurse discusses this assessment and concern with the physician, suggesting the patient be referred to the health education center.

Upon referral, the health education coordinator interviews the patient to assess learning needs and determines appropriate teaching strategies. The coordinator may actually perform the patient/family teaching or may assist the responsible nurse in incorporating appropriate teaching strategies into the patient's plan for care. The responsible nurse will then continue to follow up on the effectiveness of the teaching strategies, calling on the health education coordinator if further consultation is needed.

An additional fee is charged if the coordinator actually does patient teaching. Included in this service is a follow-up telephone call made by the coordinator to the patient after discharge. The patient's progress is then reported to the responsible nurse.

Nurses often refer patients who have multiple problems or need teaching in an uninterrupted block of time to the health education coordinator. Examples of types of patients who may be referred are diabetic patients who have ·' vision problems or hypertensive patients who speak only Spanish.

Use of the health education coordinator assists the responsible nurse in increasing his or her teaching capabilities and provides the patient who has special needs with a comprehensive and personalized teaching plan.

Besides patient teaching, health education provides other services. One emphasis in the department is on providing the community and selected industries with preventative health care courses. These courses include diet and nutrition, exercise, parenting, care of the newborn, and others.

Another emphasis is on providing information and classes for our own employees, as part of their employee benefits. The classes are offered several times a year and are held days and evenings. These courses are either free to employees or are partially paid for by the hospital. Topics include exercise for fun and health, dance-er-cise, stress management, and nutrition for over eaters. These classes are meant to help employees maintain optimal physical and mental health.

## COMMITTEE ACTIVITY

We have commented that much of the El Camino Hospital nursing organization's work is accomplished in committees. Staff development instructors provide leadership and clinical expertise in the work of several of these. In support of the philosophy of decentralization, the process of chairing committees is being passed from staff development instructors to head nurses and staff nurses. The following are some of the standing committees in which staff development instructors participate:

Staff development instructors attend medical staff committee meetings to give nursing input and assist with problem solving. Nursing committees which staff development representatives attend include Nursing Management Council, Executive Nursing Committee, Procedures Committee, and Care Planning Committee. In these committees, instructors function as educational advisors. The CPR Committee is a multidisciplinary committee that critiques Code CPRs, makes recommendations for educational needs as well as changes in CPR team composition, equipment, medications, and protocols; instructors represent nursing and education on this committee.

Staff development provides leadership for the Resource Nurse Support Committees and the Nursing Practice Committee.

## SUMMARY

The role of staff development or education in any nursing organization is to maintain and upgrade the skills of nurses in order to protect patients and provide for their quality care. In our decentralized structure we have gone beyond that, encouraging nurses' growth and development both as professionals and as people. Educators encourage nurses to become true patient advocates, to make decisions in the best interests of their patients.

To support the philosophy of decentralization, instructors have provided an assortment of educational opportunities and experiences. Being responsible and having authority to act reflects one's own responsibility for learning. Self-paced learning and a learning center are valuable assets for a decentralized structure. Leadership development has become vital for primary decision makers at all levels.

The job of the educator/instructor is never complete. New nurses continue to enter the organization, and others move into leadership positions. As the nurses at the bedside become more autonomous, they assist their new colleagues in greater proficiency within the decentralized nursing structure. In our organization, nurses do have the opportunity to grow, to learn, and to participate. And it is our belief that El Camino patients do receive better care.

# 7

## Perceptions: Views From Within

Decentralization has been at El Camino now for more than half a decade. Some members of the hospital's nursing staff have known no other system, while others have seen the hospital operate under both kinds of nursing structures. Both groups regard decentralization as a "good" word, signifying a modern, progressive method of operating the hospital nursing service. Beyond that, a definitive understanding of decentralization is less certain.

It is natural, then, to ask what decentralization actually means to those who are involved in making it operate. What is "better" about decentralization? What's it all about, really?

The hospital's nurses know what decentralization does: It makes a difference in the way they work. But their individual interpretations of that difference are interesting.

In seeking individual perceptions of decentralization it also is necessary to observe that the nature of the new organization divides the nursing staff at El Camino into two different groups. One is the line staff, those personnel who have direct responsibility for patients and patient care. The other is the support staff (coordinators and staff development personnel), none of whom is responsible for rendering direct patient care, but all of whom are important in seeing that support is always available for line personnel.

That support may come in many forms. Highly visible are the staff development personnel who provide clinical assistance, unit instructional programs, hospitalwide instructional programs, and learning center materials. Nearly as visible are the evening and night coordinators who support and assist the staff nurses of their respective shifts in management, administration and patient care matters. Less visible but no less important are other support staff, such as the quality assurance coordinator and the interdepartmental liaison coordinator, who provide services needed by the entire nursing staff.

The difference between line staff and support staff may seem slight, but it is quite important. The line staff is faced with day-to-day decision making and responsibility. It must take action every day to be certain the individual patient gets what he or she needs to recover health. For the support staff, however, there is a different kind of decision-action-resolution process. Like the general staff of an army, it must plan, provide, study and prepare, knowing it will effect action only *indirectly.* Thus its perspective is different.

A third point of view is represented by the four authors of this book. For the past two years they have immersed themselves in the details, philosophy, history, and process of decentralization. In many ways their involvement has been more intense than that of either line or support staffs. Certainly it has provided them with a viewpoint different from either of the other two groups.

For that reason it seems logical to view decentralization and its effects from all three perspectives. It also seems to be in order to give some background of the authors and how this book came to be written.

The idea for the book was generated at a Management Council meeting several years ago. Shortly afterward, a brief item appeared in the *Green Sheet,* the nursing service's weekly newsletter, asking for "anyone interested in writing a book about El Camino and decentralization to contact the nursing office." Five nurses answered the request. Four of them ultimately became the authors of *Nursing Decentralization: The El Camino Experience.* The four represent an interesting cross-section:

*Pat Pierce* is an RN who worked as a staff nurse and a supervisor under the traditional nursing system. At the time decentralization began, she was working part time in Emergency and going to school. Today she is a nurse-member of the management engineering staff assisting with the computerized medical information system.

*Nancy Hardyck* began her work at El Camino as a staff nurse in the Intensive Care Unit. She started the health service and then became a nursing supervisor under the traditional organizational structure. A major focus of her job was to interface with other hospital departments. Through this experience she had a chance to expand and give her role visibility. She was intimately involved in the organization of the new nursing structure and in the change from traditional to decentralized nursing. Today she is the nursing coordinator for interdepartmental liaison.

*Joan Althaus* started service at El Camino as a staff nurse in the Intensive Care Unit. After working full time in this area for several years, she decided to work part time while teaching and studying for her doctorate.

*Marilyn Rodgers* came to El Camino as a new graduate RN. She worked as a staff nurse and then as a charge nurse on several units until she became the first staff development instructor on the night shift. She was a member of staff development during the change to decentralization.

Taken collectively, the views of the line and support staff combined with those of the four authors represent a wide range of experience and provide insight from a variety of perceptions. In some cases these views are held in common, but in others they are not. All are presented here in an attempt to point out that decentralization will be viewed from a number of perspectives among the nursing staff. Decentralization will provide a variety of experiences as it evolves within the walls of a hospital, and it is helpful for the nursing staff to realize this fact and work with it.

Not every hospital will follow all the common threads that have appeared at El Camino. Each hospital is unique, and it is the nature of decentralization to be shaped and fitted to the circumstances that arise. In this chapter, we will show how change is perceived and examine some of the things that have transpired since our own decentralization movement began.

Above all, decentralization does bring change, and often the change is not what its planners anticipate. Sometimes it is surprising; always it is interesting. Decentralization requires creativity and self-actualization on the part of its participants, so its direction is always unique. In the long run El Camino's experience has been positive.

Bearing this in mind, let's now take an in-depth look at the effects of decentralization from the standpoints of these three groups: the line staff, the support staff, and the authors.

## REFLECTIONS FROM THE LINE STAFF

In gathering the information for this section, head nurses and staff nurses were grouped together, and their views are identified as staff nurse unless the head-nurse responses differ significantly.

A clear consequence of decentralization for line staff is elevated self-esteem. The increase in responsibility and accountability offered by the system makes staff nurses acutely aware of their individual contribution to the unit in which they serve. For the nurse who likes this kind of responsibility, it is a rewarding experience. The nurse who does not will usually seek employment elsewhere. Those who remain are willing to give more, and they show an increased loyalty to their unit and its head nurse.

Indeed, as decentralization intends, the head nurse is the central figure. The increased emphasis on budgeting and staffing at the unit level makes it almost impossible for the focus to be elsewhere.

It is surprising how rapidly individual staff nurses perceive the difference and how their relationship with the head nurse and the unit evolves. Ask staff nurses about this and they reply, "We now do budgeting at a unit level!" Or, "We have participative management!"

All levels of nursing personnel from director to nursing assistant understand that there is more authority and decision making at the unit level. This identification with the head nurse is accompanied by the staff nurses' growing perception of themselves as important. Staff nurses learn to think about and act for "their" patients, and they realize that because the supervisors and assistant directors are no longer present, a minimum of distance exists between them and the director of nursing.

This emerging individuality is accompanied by a growing interest in professional advancement. To better carry out their responsibilities—now that they are more accountable—staff nurses see clearly their need for staff development.

El Camino's nursing service boasts a high percentage of RNs—in fact, RNs comprise more than 75 percent of the nursing staff, a reflection of our emphasis on skill and responsibility. The actual breakdown by job classification as of September 1980, was 488 registered nurses (76 percent), 22 licensed vocational nurses (3 percent), 82 nursing assistants (13 percent), and 53 clinical unit secretaries (8 percent).

One result of individual involvement, improved self-esteem, and communication has been a high staff retention rate. Because individual nurses derive personal satisfaction from the system, they feel a commitment to it and are reluctant to leave. As one staff nurse puts it, "El Camino is a unique place to work. No other hospital revolves around its nurses as does this hospital." Another says, "Everyone seems happier at El Camino. This is a family style hospital. People care about one another."

Undoubtedly the emphasis on unit and individual responsibility fosters better human relationships. Staff nurses feel more important if they believe they are more involved in how the unit is run. They achieve a sense of belonging, not just to a hospital but to a specific place and a specific group of nurses—their "family," as it were.

Communication is also affected. In the traditional system, communication moves from the top down or from the bottom up through successive layers of supervising nurses. The upward movement of requests is balanced by a downward movement of orders.

In decentralization this does not happen. Communication seems to be spread in all directions, originating at all levels. An increased emphasis on communication within units is accompanied by a decrease in communication between units.

At the same time, concentration on the unit has greatly increased the burden of work for the head nurse. Much of the administrative burden once borne by supervisors and their assistants now falls on the shoulders of the head nurse. One staff nurse estimates that her head nurse is either away from the unit or involved in administrative tasks at least 60 percent of the time. While other units may not report this high a percentage of administrative work, few head nurses would deny that they do spend much more of their time pursuing details formerly dealt with outside the unit.

The head nurse has become the administrative hub of the hospital. This is evident not only to head nurses themselves, but also to staff nurses, aides, and licensed vocational nurses (LVNs). It is to the head nurse that staff nurses in units turn when they want assistance. Even though support staff exists, the natural route for finding it seems to be through the head nurse. The effect of these changes is typified by one head nurse's comment: "It sometimes gets very frustrating because the buck *does* stop here!"

Thus the degree of a unit's success and the height (or depth) of its morale is greatly dependent on the ability of its head nurse. Some staff nurses worry that decentralization has merely created a series of new supervisory positions at a slightly lower level than those eliminated along with the traditional system. It is perhaps too early to tell if this danger is more imaginary than real, but at least the potential is recognized.

Some nurses have suggested that day shifts need assistant head nurses to relieve head nurses of some of this burden. At present, a few units do have assistant head nurses on the day shift. To preclude the addition of another administrative layer between staff nurses and the director, no new positions were created for the day shift when decentralization was established. How this problem will be solved in the future remains undefined.

Another issue of concern to staff nurses is the fact that fewer resources, such as staff development and medical information system training, are available to the evening and night shifts than to those who work days. While the requirements for support are just as great—or greater—during these parts of the nursing day, it is true that fewer coordinators are available then. Some way of ensuring adequate resources for the evening and night shifts seems necessary.

Staff nurses also complain at times about the emphasis on budgeting. Because the budget has become the responsibility of the head nurse, and because budgets are now initiated at the unit level, it is natural that more emphasis exists on the budget within the unit.

Staff nurses have become aware that almost every aspect of patient care in some way is affected by the unit's budget; even so, they become tired of hearing about it. Because most staff nurses have been exposed only recently to the relationship between productivity goals, acuity ratings, the core staffing pattern, and their own workload, they are just beginning to think of these things in terms of cost. While once it was simply a matter of giving care and not paying much attention to the cost, now nurses are discovering that quality care costs money. Many nurses welcome the challenge with an increased personal interest in budgeting, developing genuine pride in how well their unit works and how successful it is in reaching or surpassing its productivity goal. But others do not share this insight into the relationship between productivity and cost. More time needs to be spent in increasing this understanding.

Administrative time for head nurses is another area that is not always clear to staff nurses. This is the time code used for administrative tasks such as scheduling and meetings, as compared to that used for patient care responsibilities. This situation is being clarified by allowing staff nurses to use administrative time for their own work on committees. In the past, staff nurses would do committee work without pay. The sanctioned use of administrative time by staff nurses underscores the importance of their input and the value of their presence to others. As we have pointed out in earlier chapters, staff nurses are now an important force on a number of standing committees within the nursing service.


## REFLECTIONS FROM THE SUPPORT STAFF

Members of the support staff are in a much better position to see the overall style and quality of interaction among various groups in the nursing service. They enjoy this vantage point because daily they meet and communicate with members of different nursing units as well as with administration. This involvement exists on many levels and can result in frustration, because there is awareness of the total picture but limited authority for direct action. This frustration was an unexpected result of the move to decentralization, and may have been caused by the gap between intellectual knowledge and personal experience.

All of El Camino's support staff members had actual clinical experience before moving into their present duties. Therefore each has a first-hand understanding of what it means to be involved in direct patient relations. The nature of their jobs requires additional and specific knowledge about the overall operation of the system. Because support staff members do not belong to any one unit, they do not have the line-staff type of unit loyalty. Their loyalty is toward the director of nursing and the hospital itself. What they have to say is crucial because it concerns the function of the system as a whole entity.

Support staff members look as much to the future as to the present, especially in their continuing concern for communication not only within and among units, but also between units and themselves. They ponder the problem of units becoming so internally loyal to the head nurse that they isolate themselves from other units and nurses.

"There's a tendency for the staff to be concerned only with their own little world," according to one support staff member. "They need to see the more global aspect of the nursing service and their part in it."

This points to an increased need for better communication. "It's a continuous problem. Sometimes the right hand doesn't know what the left hand is doing. This can lead to needless duplication of effort."

On the other hand, unit loyalty gives many nurses a place and a group with which to identify themselves. Under traditional nursing systems nurses are often shifted about, separated from authority, and removed from the sense of belonging to anything except the nursing service. This leads to low morale and high staff turnover.

El Camino nurses now have collegial relationships with other members of their unit. They are able to develop and maintain stable friendships and working arrangements, and their relationships with patients are certainly more holistic than under the traditional system of nursing organization. As a result of these relationships and feelings, moving to another hospital may be traumatic. "A nurse leaving El Camino is likely to suffer from culture shock," one support staff member says. "She's so used to unit autonomy and looking to the head nurse, she is going to face considerable readjustment in another system."

Support staff members tend to share a unique frustration over their influence on the system. It seems clear many of them miss the day-to-day contact they once had with patients. Also, realizing that their mission is to be supportive and not directive, they wish they had more to say about how things are done. In part this may be because they can see what could be done with the information they gather, and in part it may be because they do not have direct line power to affect the way in which the information is used.

As one of them says, "It is much more difficult to find job satisfaction in an advisory role. The gratification is in being responsible for getting the job done, not in telling someone how it ought to be accomplished." At the same time, support staff members see that participative management and planning is one of the strengths of decentralization. They realize that more nurses are involved in more activities than ever before—a multitude of task forces and committees seem to be constantly at work.

These feelings about job satisfaction and gratification reflect recognition of several types of power. One type, of course, is the power over people, or the "command" power. A more subtle and possibly stronger type of power is power working *through* people: a collegial power. In this usage, support people learn to make their knowledge and expertise available to the line people in such a way that they receive satisfaction from seeing their ideas used and watching others grow. At the same time, line people gain gratification from growing and seeing the results of their interest and participation in action.

Greater participation naturally leads to more results. Support staff members point out, however, that these results also require more time. "It takes a long time to get a job done because of the number of people involved," one support staff member says. "More people have input into the decision-making process."

Consensus decision making is frustrating at times; however, we consider the time well-spent. As people develop a greater understanding of this decision-making process, perhaps they will be less frustrated. There is a theory which states that if more time is invested in the initial planning and organization of a proposed change, less time will be needed for its implementation. A little retrospection will show that this theory is proving to be valid in our nursing organization. Time is taken to ensure that everyone involved in a project has a clear understanding of what needs to be accomplished, why it is needed, and how it will be done. Most projects are completed successfully because many people have been involved in the planning, development, and implementation. Participants have invested of themselves and therefore "own" part of the product.

The concept of dynamic decision making must also include a look at the people making the decisions. At El Camino, a large percentage of the nursing staff has been employed for five or more years. While any hospital would applaud such a low turnover rate, some support staff members see its inherent dangers, as well. Ideally, long-term employment and commitment should not result in stagnation and stunting of growth, but in certain situations these factors may result. Decentralization is not a static system. Its strength is dependent on each staff nurse maintaining a high level of motivation. The danger seems to have been avoided thus far, but a watchful eye should be kept open.

The support personnel agree that decentralization has caused individual staff nurses to become more aware of the need for self-improvement, particularly in professional education. This occurs because the increased individual responsibility tends to expose specific gaps in knowledge of both nursing theory and practice. As a result, staff nurses are taking advantage of many educational programs, both within the hospital and in the community.

Finally, one support staff member raises the question of whether or not decentralization is really a controllable process. Because it is constantly evolving, because it advocates and fosters change, the question of how its growth is to be controlled is an important one. Our control of the decentralization process at El Camino Hospital may parallel the control of health care by nurses.

"To the extent that we can control decentralization and move nurses into their rightful role as major influences in health care, the nursing profession will be actualized and its members will grow and contribute to patient health care goals," comments this perceptive nurse.

And this, in turn, raises a question about the direction in which decentralization is heading. In some ways it seems to have a life of its own, a condition that often diverts it from the path in which it was originally headed. It is provocative to speculate on the future of decentralization knowing that our speculations may be entirely inaccurate; ultimately, the process itself will determine its own future.

## REFLECTIONS FROM THE AUTHORS

After hearing the opinions of both line and support staff members, the authors have concluded there can exist no single definition of decentralization. Although the entire nursing staff has been touched by decentralization, it has produced different reactions in different people. Most of these reactions have been positive.

One overwhelmingly positive reaction is the increased self-esteem with which both line and support nurses view themselves. Clearly, members of the staff believe their opinions are significant; they know they are important and the work they are doing is valuable not only to themselves, but to others.

Nurses are no longer servants. They are active partners in the task of caring for the sick and in bringing about recovery. They like what they are doing. They aspire to still greater self-esteem and personal satisfaction. More and more, nurses at El Camino are speaking up, assuming authority, and becoming independent in thought and action. More and more, too, they seem ready to accept change. Just as they express a continuing loyalty to the process of decentralization, so do they realize that it will mean change—not only as it has been in the past, but also as it will be in the future.

These changes comprise an aspect of the decentralization process that seems almost contagious. Each level must self-actualize in order to meet the expectations of the adjacent vertical level. Because it looks like fun and seems effective, people seem to take to it easily.

One of the basic precepts of decentralization is the diffusion of power. In moving from a traditional to decentralized system, if a person holding power is not willing to share it and let it pass, true decentralization will either not occur or occur only with great trauma to all concerned. People who are in touch with their own inner strengths can accomplish many things, if allowed. Hidden agenda or double messages are not effective ways of dealing with such a group.

At El Camino Hospital, no one wants to return to a pre-decentralized environment. Staff members seem universally committed to the present system, realizing that the new shape of the nursing service is not a permanent one, but rather one that is still evolving. Wherever nurses suggest changes in the system, they seem careful to explain that they want only to change features, not the whole system.

Those who have been dissatisfied with the philosophy of decentralization have gone elsewhere. Those who remain do not want to leave. Although they periodically voice complaints about the need for better pay, few El Camino nurses are ready to give up the advantages of decentralization and move to a hospital where the traditional system of nursing still exists.

This increased stability has benefitted the growth of decentralization, providing continuity and familiarity with the skills and individuals on whom the system must depend. Another plus is that low turnover has decreased our orientation and training costs. On the negative side, we must consider the long-term effects of stability. If the nursing service becomes *too* stable, it may also lose its innovative potential. If it resists change, it may subvert one of the basic tenets of decentralization.

Lengthy exposure to decentralization may produce nurses incapable of working well in a traditional system. This premise has never been tested, but it implies that after assuming personal responsibility for an extended period of time a nurse may find it difficult—perhaps impossible—to work where such freedom does not exist. But this is a minor consideration today. At El

Camino, decentralization has been successful: it has constructed a system accepted and copied elsewhere.

The morale of the nursing service is high, and there is a healthy rivalry between units. El Camino is a nurse-oriented hospital. Nurses tend to support one another and to take pride in the nursing service as a whole. Certainly they are loyal to and proud of their individual units.

The authors agree that some areas need improvement. For instance, staff nurses have begun to complain about less slack time during their shifts. Slack time is the term for those few minutes here and there when nurses can sit down and reorganize their priorities, review cases under their control, and talk informally without demands on time or attention. It used to be present because productivity wasn't as closely controlled. Now that census and staffing are more closely correlated, shifts don't vary so much in workload per nurse.

One method of overcoming this problem may be better time management. Time management is now part of the MOD program being offered to assistant head nurses as well as head nurses and management personnel. It seems reasonable to expect that as their time management knowledge increases, assistant head nurses may be able to share their knowledge with staff nurses, and more time may be created for use as the staff nurse desires.

Another problem with which head nurses must contend is the unit's core curriculum, the set of specific procedures that each nurse in a given unit is expected to learn and know. When new nurses are hired, they are assessed for their knowledge of the unit's core curriculum, and individual plans are developed to correct their deficiencies. Some nurses who were at El Camino before decentralization tend to resist head nurses' requests to update deficiencies. Perhaps there has been insufficient time allotted for the idea to spread throughout all personnel. Since this idea is quite innovative, it may just take longer to fully implement—like decentralization itself.

Writing nursing care plans is another area where compliance lagged but has now increased. Staff development presented many classes and workshops on care-plan writing, but somehow the staff nurses did not appear motivated to write them on all patients. As the director placed more emphasis on this area and the head nurses included care-plan writing in staff nurse evaluations, the situation improved. However, what helped most was the creation of the Care Planning Committee, comprised of staff representation from all units. Operating with truly democratic input and feedback, the committee was given power to change care-plan formats on a hospitalwide basis as it saw fit. Because staff nurses were delegated this responsibility and accountability for their actions, care plans are now being written.

Another successful effort dealt with the problem of float nurses. Although floats have been reduced to a minimum at El Camino, a few are necessary. With the development of decentralization and the disappearance of the central nursing office, floats became essentially homeless. For a time they were assigned to the complexes, but this still left them without a sense of belonging to anyone. The solution has been to assign floats to individual head nurses. This permits them to get information, support, and evaluations from a specific person.

Decentralization has evoked an interest in lateral promotion, working toward increased skills while remaining in the same job. The concept of lateral promotion means additional pay or differential, but it is seen as a positive outgrowth of decentralization. Job sharing and job exchanges are ways to facilitate lateral interchange. Learning someone else's job—even learning their circumstances of work—can be educational.

One final complaint sometimes is heard from the nursing service: "If we are the state-of-the-art, why aren't we more perfect?"

The answer to this question lies in the answer to the question of individual self-esteem and sense of worth. Decentralization is a system that works best for the individual who is self-motivated. The inner direction of self is important in an organization where worth, effort, and decision making arise from how well or how poorly the individual responds to challenges. Those who tend to seek the answers to challenge from others, from the organization or unit, or from some other area outside themselves, do not do as well as the inner-directed. Decentralization tends to weed such individuals from the ranks of the nursing service and to replace them with those who like independence, freedom, the assumption of responsibility, and the willingness to be accountable. Our degree of perfection, then, is dependent on the capabilities and the self-motivation of the staff.

With all its problems and with its continual self-examination, decentralization *is* working. It is working because it invites all nurses to be a part of it, and the very essence of decentralization is the necessity of working through people. It fosters professional improvement, it enhances self-esteem, it helps to place nurses on a more equal footing with physicians. It attracts those who have high levels of skill, good motivation, plus an interest in learning, growing, giving, and being heard. All these qualities can be summed up in the term "self-actualization," something that decentralization both provides and thrives on. Its concept involves the letting go of predetermined roles and the defining of personal preferences and abilities. It involves relinquishing power from a few to many until it becomes diffused. It requires confident individuals who find security within themselves rather than in the sameness of their functions. Each decentralized hospital will be a self-designed organization that uses the unique abilities of its members in new and creative ways. It will be a truly "organic" organization that can never be duplicated and that continues to change with the cycle of its human members.

Decentralization is not without imperfections, but it is a system that constantly seeks to convert its problems into improvements. It is neither rigid nor bound by dogma. It is conceived and constructed in the belief that change is necessary.

In this sense, it is an empirical system, one in which the questions most often asked are "Does it work? And if it does not, how can it be made to work?"

After spending two years looking closely and carefully at decentralization from every possible point of view, we are ready to say, "Yes, decentralization is working. It is working for us. *We believe it can work for you, too!*"

# 8

---

# *Future Fantasy: Through the Medicine Glass*

In the past seven chapters, we have defined, described, and analyzed the realities of our successful decentralized nursing organization. While reviewing the past and considering the present, we also fantasized about the future. We want to share it with you, because it was fun!

Come dream with us . . .

" . . . Where am I?" Alice asked, sitting up and rubbing her eyes. The room was white, barren, silent, and empty except for one other young woman, who sat at the console of a computer terminal. Alice could not see her very distinctly at first. She rubbed her eyes again and the young woman became more visible.

"Don't you remember?"

After a moment it began to come back to Alice. She had been sitting in an easy chair in front of the television set.

"I must have fallen asleep," she said.

"It's hard to dream without falling asleep," responded the other young woman.

"I *am* dreaming!" Alice announced.

"I certainly hope so," the young woman said dryly.

Alice got up out of her chair, and it immediately disappeared. Her feet seemed steady enough, although she felt she was moving rather slowly, almost as if she were . . . well, in a dream.

"If you're a figment of my imagination, you must have a name," she observed aloud.

"Sure. Don't you remember? I'm Alicia. You used to see me a lot when you were little. I'm what you are going to be in the future."

"Really?" said Alice. "How enchanting. An alter ego."

"I don't know about your ego. That's for psychiatrists to look into," Alicia said. "I can only show you around the hospital."

"That's very nice of you."

"It's nothing any alter ego wouldn't do."

"You don't have to be unpleasant about it," ventured Alice, still quite confused.

"I'm not being unpleasant. I just don't like working after so long a time off. It's a lot of trouble, you know, running around getting a dream together."

"I'm sure it is," Alice sympathized, "and I appreciate your being here." (At this point she decided it would be a good idea to change the subject.) "This seems like a nice place to work."

"The dream or the hospital?"

"I meant the hospital."

"It is," replied the mysterious Alicia. "That's the best part of a dream. Everyone is nice and things work the way they should. You can go exactly where you want to go and see exactly what you want to see."

"I really would like to look around," Alice said. "This looks like the hospital where I work . . . or is it *worked?*"

"Well, it is . . . and it was, too. We are in the same place, but the time is in your future."

Alice had a sudden thought: "This hospital still has a decentralized nursing organization, doesn't it?"

"Certainly. Not only that, but the whole health care system is 'decentralized.' Health care and prevention are accomplished by teams of health professionals and the patient—or 'client'—is considered an equal member of the team. Now what would you like to see?" Alicia tapped her fingers with some impatience on the edge of her console.

"Well, first I'd like to see what the front of the hospital looks like."

"Very well," Alicia said. "That's easy enough. It really doesn't look much different today than it did years ago." She punched two keys on the computer terminal and slowly the room around them grew hazy. Then, at the far wall, the haze ran together, became fixed, and turned into a picture. Actually, it seemed more than a picture, as if the room had opened and they were looking out the open end. The hospital buildings stood there, just as Alice remembered them. For a moment she thought she was wide awake and not dreaming after all.

"Somehow I expected something different. It looks just the same." "I told you it was," Alicia said reprovingly. "It's different here and there. See, there are solar panels on the roof now to generate heat and electricity—and those are electric transit vehicles down there on the road. Otherwise it looks much the same. They don't build hospitals like this anymore. It's much too expensive, so they do everything they can to use existing hospitals. But don't be disappointed. There *are* a whole lot of differences, all on the inside.

"Hospitals have agreed to create specialized regional care centers. They are established with the special needs of the local community in mind. Radiotherapy is an example. The cost of equipment is phenomenal, and our Health

Systems Agency has not been willing to approve duplication at different facilities. The radiotherapy center is in a hospital about ten miles from here. Nearby, in another hospital, there is a chemotherapy center. Since interferon has been used so extensively, chemotherapy has grown by leaps and bounds. Many cancer patients go there, both from here and other hospitals. We have become a cardiac care center. We see more heart patients, and the other hospitals see more patients in their specialities—it all evens out in the long run."

"Can I see *anything* I want?" Alice said.

"In a dream you can see anything you want to—and some things you don't want to," Alicia replied. "You just have to tell me what it is you want."

"Well," said Alice, after a little reflection, "I'd like to see what a nurse looks like now."

"First of all, we don't call them nurses anymore," Alicia said. "That's a sexist description of an occupation."

"Excuse me," said Alice. "What *do* you call them?"

"Well, there are lots of health facilitators who work here now. And then there are the health care associates . . . "

Alice wrinkled her nose, but out of courtesy said nothing.

Alicia manipulated her keyboard. "There . . . "(A young woman appeared in the display in place of the hospital.) "That's a health care facilitator."

"She's not wearing a uniform!"

"Uniforms were on their way out even when you were a nurse. Health care facilitators wear uniforms about as often as doctors do—when it's necessary to keep clean, mostly."

"But they used to tell us we didn't look professional if we didn't wear a uniform!"

"Professional *is* as professional *does,*" Alicia declared with a smile at her dreamlike attempt at humor. "Health care facilitators are professionals who give health care. Sometimes they get paid by the case, sometimes they contract with the hospital to provide certain skills. Often, they care for their clients in private offices. Some of them are employed directly by hospitals. However they work, the bill for their assistance is separate and what their services cost can be easily identified! The hospital's bill reflects things like food and room charges and clerical services, all separately from health facilitation and health associate services. But the most important thing is the change in the emphasis of their care."

"What do you mean?"

"Well, they are truly 'wellness enhancers.' They facilitate health by disease prevention and are as much interested in preventing people from going to the hospital as they are in taking care of them after they get admitted. They are also closely involved with transition from home to hospital and back again. Our large elderly population especially needs this service.

"The patient's health facilitator sometimes visits the home and the home-care facilitator may visit the patient in the hospital, depending on individual needs. There is careful attention to the liaison to ensure continuity of excellent quality care for the patient. Care *is* taken not to duplicate services. There is a place in patient care for machines, but that is only a short-term need. After the acute phase is past, then people have to take over!"

Alicia had begun to sound a bit like a textbook, but her enthusiasm was contagious. "The continuing care center is another example of changing concepts of care. It is especially pertinent to the needs of the elderly. Since they generally need more help during convalescence but don't need acute, intensive nursing care, they use the continuing care center sometimes as a day center, sometimes for 24-hour care in the transition to normal life after illness."

Alice clapped her hands. "It all sounds wonderful!" she exclaimed. "And what are the facilitators *paid* for all these services?"

"Well," Alicia said, "they have a lot of added new responsibilities and independence . . . and they also have equal status with the medical profession. Health facilitators' incomes vary quite a bit, because what they make is determined by how much energy and skill they possess. They are mainly independent operators in a free market. A good health facilitator who carries a full practice makes much more than a nurse used to.

"I also have to explain, because it is hard to show it with the computer, that they work in a much different way than they did when you were a . . . er . . . nurse."

"How?" Alice asked.

"It's been possible to eliminate much of the old, fixed, three-shift eight-hour days."

"I never thought *that* would happen."

"Well, it didn't happen overnight. But gradually, partly through the contractual system and individual initiative, health facilitators have changed the way sick people are cared for."

"And it's still possible to cover 24 hours in the acute care hospital?"

"Lots of things are done to lower staffing requirements," explained Alicia. "It's now possible to predict the types of patients and the patient load we can expect. Research has shown that certain illnesses occur at specific seasons. There are also external factors that influence admissions—medical conventions, temporary changes in local employment patterns, and so on. This gives us a very accurate picture of what to expect on both short- and long-term projections. Operating room and associated schedules are controlled so that greatest need for staff occurs when it is available. Only long-term patients stay here over weekends, and there are significantly fewer of them than before. There are more one-day procedures and patients clustered on units according to length of stay, so that units do not function seven days a week or even 24 hours a day. Our sophisticated life-system monitors require fewer staff for acute care. And people come to the hospital to stay a lot less often than they used to, so the need for 24-hour coverage has decreased in volume."

"We have fine staffing schedules made up by this." Alicia tapped the computer almost affectionately with the palm of her hand. Then she smiled for the first time. It was the sort of dazzling smile one might reserve for a respected colleague, indeed Alicia thought of the computer as being almost human. Realizing this, Alice wondered if she had a name for it, like Hal or Charlie, or something like that, but she decided she had better not ask. Suddenly she felt old and obsolete.

"I suppose it can tell me how many sick hours I have left, and my biorhythms for today, and what kind of man I'm likely to marry."

"Almost. Your dream isn't long enough to tell you about all the things the computer can do for you, but let me make a stab at it." She took a deep breath:

"As care plans are built for patients, acuities are extracted from plans. The system is based on a highly refined scoring system begun years ago. The scoring system takes into consideration all aspects of patient care. This includes emotional support and teaching, as well as the more task-oriented chores. The integration of these more subtle, yet indispensible aspects of total patient care into the acuity system is a major accomplishment!

"These patient care requirements can be matched to the staff available and patient loads projected. It can tell you what your skills are and what they should be for any patient in this hospital! It keeps a profile of how well you are handling your patients and tells you if you could be doing a better job! It can tell you how many patients you are likely to have in the Trauma Department next weekend and if you'll need extra health facilitators to care for them. It can monitor the life systems of every patient in the hospital . . . "

She paused for breath.

"Wait a minute, wait a minute!" Alice interrupted, seizing the moment. "Run that last one by me again."

"I said the computer can help monitor every patient in the hospital, 24 hours a day."

"Show me."

"Certainly."

Alicia's hands danced over the keyboard and a man appeared at the end of the room, walking away from them down the corridor.

"Who's that?"

"It's a patient, Mr. Anton. He's coming into the hospital to have his gallbladder removed. His regular health facilitator at the Health Promotion Center referred him to the surgeon, and she has been working with both of them to prepare Mr. Anton for surgery. She will take over his home care from the acute care facilitator after he is stabilized at home."

The man entered what Alice recognized as the hospital lobby and went to a directory board.

"What's he doing?"

"He's come to pick out his health facilitator."

"You mean he's actually going to pick his own nurse?"

" . . . health facilitator, *please*. Yes, more or less. What's so radical about that? Patients picked their own doctors in 1980. It was only a matter of time before they expected to select their health facilitators as well. Sometimes the computer matches a facilitator who has certain skills with a patient who has certain needs. Since Mr. Anton's case is relatively simple, he is going to use the facilitator who cared for him last year when he had a carotid bypass. His regular health facilitator advised him in this decision, but he is free to request a computer match or choose whomever he wants."

"My," was all Alice could think of to say.

She watched as Mr. Anton, having located the health facilitator group he wanted, walked down the hall to the office and went inside. A facilitator— Alice found she could think facilitator instead of *nurse* now and then—seated him, typed his description and other information into a computer terminal, and then snapped a small metal bracelet around his wrist.

"Is that his identification bracelet?"

"It's more than that. It's also his telemetry monitor. It records his vital signs continuously while he's ambulatory. Now look . . . "

Alicia had brought up another picture for display. The patient had materialized in a bed. A large thin metallic band hung on the wall behind him.

"What's that?" Alice asked.

"That band is placed around Mr. Anton's chest just prior to surgery. It's just a more sophisticated set of sensors, and he'll wear it until he's ambulatory again. It's comfortable enough so that he won't notice it, and meantime it will keep the monitoring center right up to the minute on how he's doing."

"He can't talk through it can he?"

"As a matter of fact, he can. He doesn't need a call button when he wants help. He can actuate his communicator."

"What's a communicator?"

"I'd forgotten how long you'd been asleep," Alicia said. "Everyone's got a communicator." She held her own up. It looked much like a digital wristwatch. "See, the nurse . . . er . . . facilitator has one, too."

"I've often wished I had one instead of listening to the page system," Alice said.

"It's one of the handiest inventions in communication," Alicia said with feeling. "We can actually input and output some information from the medical information system through the ones we wear."

"That's certainly more than Dick Tracy's wrist radio could do," Alice said.

"Who?" Alicia frowned.

"Never mind. It was before your time."

"I could try the memory bank in the computer." Alicia seemed curious.

"As you said, this dream isn't long enough. There's a lot more I'd like to see, anyway," urged Alice, conscious of all she wanted to absorb.

A woman had entered the picture and was talking to the patient.

"Who's that?"

"She's the doctor come to see Mr. Anton." The doctor raised her wrist and began talking into her communicator.

"What's she doing?"

"Making some notes, I expect. The health facilitator is giving her some history and personal information. And it looks like she's giving some orders."

"*She's* giving the *doctor* orders?"

"Maybe 'orders' is the wrong word. She's telling the doctor what the health care plan for the patient entails, so they can cooperate on planning the surgery and the care that comes afterward. The computer prints out a complete patient profile on request, with all the documented plans and data regarding his physical condition. These days health facilitators work with doctors on a collegial basis. The MD will also discuss the medical care plan with her and they will work with the patient, initially. Later on, other members of the health care team may be brought in as necessary."

"I wouldn't have believed it if I hadn't seen it!"

"Yes, it's really great that the days when doctors were *bothered* by nursing interventions are over! These days most doctors and nurses work very well together, and many other health professionals are also included with equal status on the care team. All the health care givers follow the same education ladders in school, you know."

"You mean nurses go to medical school?"

"Sort of. That is, not exactly. But then doctors don't go to medical school either, anymore."

Alicia's computer screen displayed a diagram. "This is the career ladder for health professionals. Notice that everyone, including physicians, health facilitators, pharmacists, and dietitians get the same basic education."

"Kind of pre-professional curriculum?"

"Exactly. But I'd appreciate it if you didn't interrupt this dream so much. Otherwise, it will be over and you won't have seen all you want to see. Now, as I was saying, anyone entering the health care field now gets the same basic education. There is a lot more emphasis on health maintenance and disease prevention. All health professionals continue, branching into their area of specialization. Then, at various points, students have completed enough schooling to go to work at one job or another in health care; they have the option of dropping off the ladder or continuing on to a higher level of specialization. For example, there are the health care associates, who generally give direct patient care. They have health-care-associate certificates. If they want a degree in health care facilitation, they can return to school, building on the academic work they completed earlier."

"What's the difference between a nurse—that is, a health facilitator,—and a physician?"

Alicia looked at Alice intently. "That's a very good question. There isn't much difference in years of education, but there is a difference in approach. The physician is still looking at pathology, trying to cure disease after it happens. The health facilitator is looking for ways to prevent disease from happening."

"Don't any health facilitators render care to patients any more?"

"You weren't listening," Alice said a little crossly. "Of course they do. The health care associates do, too. Some health care facilitators prefer to render acute care, but the emphasis of what they do is still prevention, and they strive to give the patients control over their own illnesses rather than to generate an 'I made you well' feeling. The various types of health facilitators are like the specialities in medicine that you knew. You can pick and choose."

"But if the prevention really works, then there won't be very many sick, right?"

"Right!"

"And no one will make any money because no one will be sick."

"Very astute. But others thought of that, too. Keeping people well involves as much financial reward as caring for them after they are sick.

"That's where third-party payors and the government come in. It was a hard job, but finally they were convinced that maintaining good health is as valuable, even more valuable, than curing disease. So health-care professionals get incentives, financial ones, for *keeping* people well. They contract for health maintenance and they get cost analysis and peer review of the job they are doing. The better the job, the better the pay. It's as simple as that."

"It sounds too good to be true."

"I'll admit that it's dreamlike, but it could, like anything in a dream, become reality."

"You mean all dreams come true?"

"I can only reassure you that while they don't always, they always *can.* There's always the possibility." Alicia looked vexed again.

"Look," she continued, "I'm not going to have to spend all night shoring up your confidence, am I? Isn't there something else you'd like to see?"

"Yes, I'd like to see some more of nursing structure in the hospital. It certainly sounds as if it is even more decentralized than it was in 1980."

"It is. But I have to be sure you understand that a lot of health facilitation now takes place outside the acute-care general hospital. Health facilitators have had to reach out into the community in their attempts at disease prevention.

"A lot of it has been work on contracts between individual or group health facilitators. Some of them contract with the government. Some are with private industry. Some are with foundations and charitable organizations. Health facilitators also are involved in teaching both themselves and others. Here, look at this . . . "

The display screen showed a pleasant room with men and women gathered in conversation.

"It looks like a waiting room," Alice observed.

"That's what it is. It's in a health promotion center."

"A what?"

"A place where people can go for a variety of things designed to promote or improve their health. This one provides patient education, physical examinations, books, pamphlets, learning modules, all kinds of communicative devices. And, of course, consultations with health facilitators, if they're needed."

"That's wonderful," said Alice. "I've always wanted to work in a place like that. It's been one of my dreams."

"It certainly has," Alicia said with a smile.

Alice laughed. "You caught me there. But I don't see exactly what all this has to do with decentralization."

"I thought I was bringing you along a little too rapidly," Alicia sighed. "This facility is part of the outreach of what you used to call the 'nursing service' at your hospital. It's only one of many things they're doing these days. Operating a hospital child-care center for working parents is another. And we have several dialysis facilities that are contracting to operate a dialysis training center."

"About decentralization . . . " Alice interjected.

"All right, all right. I just thought you should appreciate the fact that health facilitators are in a lot more—and different—places than nurses used to be. In fact, nursing as a concept just isn't anymore. We owe a lot to Florence Nightingale, but she's been gone for a long time. That view of what can be done for health care is something that's in the past. We have to look forward toward a new century. It's not very far away, you know."

Alice had the weird feeling that Alicia thought of her as a Florence Nightingale type. She decided it was best not to ask again about decentralization, so she just waited.

Alicia studied the console of the computer for a moment or two and then typed a command. The image of a young man appeared. He, too, was seated at a computer terminal.

"This is a unit secretary. He's checking into the number of staff available for the coming weekend."

Alice could see figures appearing on the terminal screen.

"This is one of the important ways in which decentralization has had its effect on the hospital. All staff members have their profiles written into the computer when they are employed.

"It shows their skills, their availability, the days and hours they have worked and can work; in fact, it contains everything there is to know about them, professionally. The computer buzzes a warning when a discrepancy in available staffing and requirements is detected. Then it's up to the secretary to interpret the printout and see what the problem is. The secretary must either call in different staff, more staff, or cancel some staff. If further advice is needed, an administrative health facilitator is available."

The secretary typed a new set of instructions.

"Now he's looking at the patient acuities for the next time period," Alicia added. "That approach certainly ought to help staffing and budgeting," Alice said with admiration.

"Oh, it does, but the profiles are important for another reason. Just wait a moment."

The picture at the end of the room changed again and a woman was seated at a terminal.

"That's a health facilitator," Alicia said. "Watch."

The woman typed her name into the terminal and then selected "Skills Profile."

"What's she doing?"

"Pay attention! She's checking her computer evaluation. The system keeps track of the care given to her patients. If the patient care goals on the care plan are not met on time (which means her patients don't progress as they should), this will show on her profile. On the other hand, if she is doing well, this will show too. This evaluation is also available to the peer review committee. Specific educational programs are recommended to remedy deficiencies, if any are identified. There is a huge learning center for the county a few miles from here. Computer-assisted teaching is available. Our computer lists expert facilitators who are available to precept any of their peers who need additional support and teaching. All current education programs in the state are in the computer. A facilitator can choose a desired subject and get a list of programs scheduled on that subject."

The facilitator on the screen studied her terminal display intently. The information came up as a kind of graph. In most places the graph had two parallel lines; here and there a deviation was evident.

"She's doing alright," Alicia said. "A deficiency in neuro assessment, but it's not bad. She can get some instruction from a teaching module, or, if necessary, take some practical instruction from an expert on the subject. This kind of personal evaluation is very important and it's something that never would happen without decentralization. And without a computer, I suppose."

The health facilitator turned off the terminal, stood up, and departed down a corridor.

"Where's she going?"

Alicia retrieved a time schedule on her terminal. "It's time for the all-staff monthly meeting, I guess."

"All staff?"

"Just like physicians used to have in your day. It's one of the ways the health facilitators can improve their communication with one another.

"The administrator for health facilitation meets with the staff once a month, because she's found in spite of all the electronics there is no substitute for a face-to-face talk now and then. It's not a long meeting, but it's an important one."

Alice was silent. She could not remember a time when all staff *nurses* had gathered for a monthly meeting.

"Don't look so surprised," Alicia said. "Doctors and health facilitators have separate staff meetings most of the time, but they have equal staff privileges. A facilitator gets admitted to practice in the hospital just as a doctor does. There are credentials committees, sponsors, just as there always have been for physicians. It's a way to be sure of the quality of personnel."

"It certainly sounds like a good idea."

"It is, I think. Once a year there's a joint facilitator-physician staff meeting."

"That's hard to believe," Alice said.

"I told you this was a dream," Alicia repeated (somewhat testily, Alice thought). Alicia punched up another picture. A group of men and women were sitting in a room, drinking coffee and chatting.

"What's that?" Alice asked, although she thought she knew.

"It's the lounge."

"You mean . . . "

"That's right. It's what used to be called the doctor's lounge. Now everyone uses it. There's freedom to mix, compare notes, and work out problems in a less formal way."

Alice let out a low whistle.

"Quiet!" Alicia snapped. "Someone will think you're snoring."

Alice put her hand over her mouth. Then she took it away again. "How did it ever happen?"

"It just happened. Social integration is easy after professional integration takes place. Did you know the hospital administrator is a former health facilitator?"

"You're kidding."

"No."

Alice got a momentary glimpse of an attractive, middle-aged woman seated at a desk.

"She used to be a health facilitator. In fact, she started as a staff nurse, not long after your time. Eventually she became a facilitator and then went on to become the administrator for health facilitation. When the chance came along to take advantage of the hospital's tuition plan, she obtained additional education in medical economics. After the former administrator retired, she moved into his job; and she's doing very well."

"Did you say 'hospital tuition plan'?" Alice asked in surprise.

"The hospital pays for the education on the condition that the facilitator's skills be available to the hospital for a specific length of time. That's only fair."

"Eminently," Alice said. Then she sighed.

"What's the matter?"

"I always had the feeling I was born too early," she said.

"Well, I don't pick my alter egos, either, you know."

"You mean I should brighten the unit where I am?"

"If you want to take it that way."

Alice decided Alicia was probably right. Besides, she wanted to change the subject again. "What else have you got to show me?" she asked.

A door marked "Health Facilitation Research" appeared.

"When you were active and awake, there wasn't much research, right?"

"No, and I always wished there were more time. But then, I guess we never had the money to carry it out."

"Well, we have both, now. Today it's not uncommon for health facilitators to take time off for research projects. Here comes a researcher now. She has a grant to study better ways to bridge communication gaps occurring between health care professionals. Most facilitators take three months a year to do research. Their time is counted as productive, because they are acquiring new useful knowledge. Their salaries are paid from research funds provided by government and private foundations. New ideas have been easier to introduce when backed with good research. Health facilitators also do other kinds of research, too."

"Like what?"

Alicia produced another picture. This time it was a group of people engaged in a lively conversation. "They're discussing the effect of this year's changes in regulations for National Health Insurance," she observed.

"So it finally arrived," Alice said.

"Yes. Planning how to work with it and its regulations has been a major challenge to all hospitals. It's taken cooperation from all disciplines. They're all represented at this meeting, the ombudsman, the administrator for medical care, the administrator for health facilitation, even the staff economist. He used to be a health facilitator, too."

Alicia pushed a key on her keyboard and a small office materialized. Four people became visible, sitting around a table.

"There's Dr. McLean!" Alice exclaimed. "I know him!"

"He was just starting practice when you were there," Alicia said reassuringly.

"Who are the others?"

"Well, there's Ms. Young, the dietitian; Mr. Warling, the health facilitator; and Ms. Abrams, a patient. They're developing her health care plan together."

"That's certainly getting the patient involved in care planning," Alice said.

"It shows how important her input is in the health care picture. You'll find patients a lot less afraid to ask questions now. Sometimes it seems to me they ask too many, but that's good. It shows they are interested and confident.

They are even telling the health facilitator and the doctor what they want in the way of care."

"How do they know enough to do that? Do patients go to school, too?"

"Right. Health education has grown tremendously, not only for staff personnel, but also for patients and clients. In fact, it has become a major source of revenue for the health facilitation staff."

"Who pays for it?"

"Insurance programs mostly. They've come to realize the value of education in health care and disease prevention. And income tax deductions are allowed for those who stay healthy."

Alice tried to pinch herself to be sure that this was true, then realized it was only a dream. But Alicia was not paying any attention to her. She was still expounding the virtues of patient education:

"The classes offered cover everything from overeating to anxiety. Childbirth preparation, cooking for special diets, dealing with chronic illness, understanding one's illness, exercise classes—they're all programs available at the health promotion center. For inpatients, the computer periodically prints out lists of patients in predetermined classifications for which health education programs are available. Then special programs can be scheduled on closed-circuit television to meet the needs of the changing hospital population."

"My goodness," Alice said. "And I suppose there's a lot of emphasis on aging. I feel suddenly aged myself now that I'm older than I really am—if you know what I mean."

If Alicia thought this was funny, she didn't let on.

"Yes, we must meet the special needs of the increasing elderly population, but I think what's equally important is the growing relationship between the health facilitator and the patient. Here, let me show you."

A new picture appeared on the screen: the living room of an attractive small apartment. In it what was obviously a health facilitator was visiting with an elderly woman in a bathrobe.

"She's a patient recovering from an operation. The health facilitator took care of her while she was in the hospital, and she's been making home visits now. This lady is a widow and the personal relationship is probably as important as anything else the facilitator is doing. This client was using the human support services prior to her surgery and will continue to do so."

"Human support was fairly new in 1980," Alice remarked.

"That's right. It has come a long way from simply being of assistance in times of grief or crisis in the hospital. The human support group now offers a whole range of social services plus a discharge-planning consultant service. They support our hospital personnel, as well. People still get 'burned out' like they always have, and human support has an extensive program to help them and other hospital personnel keep healthy, happy, and on the job."

Alicia glanced at digital numbers clicking away in the corner of the display screen. "In fact," she said, "I don't have enough time left in this dream to tell you all that human support can do, but just let me say [here, Alice thought she sounded somewhat like a politician] that it is part of a program to help health care facilitators and other health professionals stay stable in what is obviously still a high-stress occupation. Even doctors attend."

"Do they have massage?" Alice asked, nervously attempting humor. "I'm beginning to feel like I had a restless night."

Alicia stared at her sternly. "We're almost through," she said. "And yes, massage therapy is available along with things like hypnosis, biofeedback, yoga, meditation therapy, and a program of earned sabbaticals."

"That's what I need," Alice sighed. "A sabbatical."

"You'll either have to stay asleep for awhile longer or wait a few more years," Alicia said primly. "The time warp you are in doesn't have them available yet."

"I could use one right now," said Alice.

Alicia regarded her quizzically. "This dream isn't turning into a nightmare, is it? What did you have to eat for supper?"

"I had scrambled eggs and toast," Alice replied. "And I'm not going to have a nightmare—I hope—it's just that there's been a lot to absorb in one evening."

"We don't have much further to go," Alicia said.

"All right, but I feel like I worked both a day and a night shift consecutively."

Alicia paid no attention to this. "Now," she went on as crisply as ever, "the biggest problem with human support programs wasn't in getting things going but in getting *payment* for them. Recognizing how valuable these services are, it's hard to understand how in your time such things weren't allowable."

Alice surpressed a yawn. She wondered how she could be sleepy while in the midst of a dream.

"You seem to be losing interest," Alicia said.

"It's not that. I think I'm beginning to wake up."

"It's just as well," remarked Alicia, glancing again at her digital real-time clock. "I've got to be going anyway. I've been commuting to the Health Facilitation Center in Boulder, Colorado, and it's time for my materialization passage. If I miss it, I won't be able to get a passage until tomorrow morning."

"Materialization?" Alice murmured somewhat foggily. She was beginning to lose focus on Alicia.

"It's faster and safer than flying," Alicia said, her businesslike voice slowly becoming fainter. "I've got a fellowship to the center. That's how I could tell you so much about all these things . . . "

"Wait a minute," Alice said, "I still have a couple of questions . . . ."

"I know. You've got a lot of them. People in real time always do. It's much easier when you're dematerialized, you know. Then the answers seem quite simple."

"But . . . " Alice started to say. "I don't know how to dematerialize . . . I've heard to decentralize everyone has to self-actualize. But *dematerialize?*"

She thought she heard the answer to that, but she wasn't sure. It seemed, as the room slowly melted around her and rearranged itself into her television set, easy chair, and apartment wall, that she heard Alicia's voice—somehow sounding much like her own—saying, " . . . but you can still dream, can't you?"

And then she woke up.

"Yes," she said to herself—and for all she knew, also to Alicia somewhere— "I surely can!"

# *Appendixes*

A   El Camino Hospital Evaluation
of Total Nursing Care

B   Guidelines for Integrating Nursing
Process into Practice

C   El Camino Hospital Flyer

D   The *Green Sheet:* Nursing
Service Update

E   New Employee Progress Evaluation

F   Hospital Organizational Chart

G   Nursing Service Annual Report 1980

H   Glossary

## Appendix A.   El Camino Hospital Evaluation of Total Nursing Care

DATE _____ UNIT _____          Patient Label
DIAGNOSIS _____
TRANSFERRED FROM _____ DATE TRANSFERRED _____
EVALUATION DONE BY _____

### I.   PHYSICAL NEEDS

#### A. Skin Integrity

| Patient Care | YES | NO | NA | Care Plan/Documentation | YES | NO | NA |
|---|---|---|---|---|---|---|---|
| 1. Clean and dry: | | | | I. Problems Identified: | | | |
| 2. Skin Dry? | | | | II. Nursing orders re: | | | |
| 3. Odor? | | | |   a. Skin Care | | | |
| 4. Reddened? | | | |   b. Decubiti prevention | | | |
| 5. Decubiti? | | | |   c. Decubiti care | | | |
| 6. Pressure areas apparent? | | | | III. Plan in current format | | | |
| 7. Rash? | | | | IV. E/O reflected in N/N | | | |

#### B. Hydration and Fluid Balance

| Patient Care | YES | NO | NA | Care Plan/Documentation | YES | NO | NA |
|---|---|---|---|---|---|---|---|
| 1. Fluid at bedside (NPO/NA) | | | | I. Problem Identified: | | | |
| 2. IV fluid: | | | | II. NO regarding: | | | |
|   a. Date and time? | | | |   a. Limit fluids | | | |
|   b. Correct fluid? | | | |   b. Encourage fluids | | | |
|   c. Correct amt. & rate? | | | |   c. IV fluids | | | |
|   d. Medication labeled? | | | | III. Plan in current format | | | |
|   e. IV red or tender? | | | | IV. E/O reflected in N/N | | | |
|   f. Tubing w/extension secured | | | | | | | |
|   g. IV site labeled with date, needle size & RN? | | | | | | | |
|   h. IV tubing & dressing changed: | | | | | | | |
|   i. Rotation of sites? | | | | | | | |
| 3. Hydration: | | | | | | | |
|   a. Limitation? | | | | | | | |
|   b. Push? | | | | | | | |
| 4. Heparin lock? | | | | | | | |
|   a. Site labeled with date, needle size and RN? | | | | | | | |

## Appendix A *(continued)*

### C. Respiratory Status

| Patient Care | YES | NO | NA | Care Plan/Documentation | YES | NO | NA |
|---|---|---|---|---|---|---|---|
| 1. Patient turns regularly? | | | | I Problem Identified | | | |
| 2. Patient supports chest, op. site when coughing? | | | | II. NO regarding: | | | |
| | | | | a. Positioning | | | |
| 3. Problems with breathing | | | | b. Turning regularly | | | |
| a. Preventive | | | | c. Deep breathing | | | |
| 4. Tracheostomy: | | | | d. Coughing | | | |
| a. Needs suctioning? | | | | e. Trach care | | | |
| b. Approp. equipment? | | | | f. Pt. teaching | | | |
| c. Humidification? | | | | g. Chest tube routine | | | |
| 5. Chest tubes patent? | | | | h. Comm. method | | | |
| a. Emergency clamp? | | | | III. Plan in current format | | | |
| 6. Suction equipment? | | | | IV. E/O reflected in N.N. | | | |
| 7. Respiratory supportive equipment? | | | | | | | |
| 8. Communication problem? | | | | | | | |

### D. Musculoskeletal Function

| Patient Care | YES | NO | NA | Care Plan/Documentation | YES | NO | NA |
|---|---|---|---|---|---|---|---|
| 1. Activity as ordered? | | | | I. Problem Identified? | | | |
| 2. Muscle conditioning? | | | | II. Nursing orders regarding: | | | |
| 3. Corrective equipment? | | | | 1. Activity (type and amount)? | | | |
| 4. Needs assistance? | | | | 2. Muscle conditioning? | | | |
| 5. Body in alignment? | | | | 3. Corrective equipment identified? | | | |
| 6. Patient knows activity Rx? | | | | 4. Number of people needed to assist patient? | | | |
| | | | | 5. Plan in correct form? | | | |
| | | | | 6. E/O reflected in N.N.? | | | |

### E. Dietary

| Patient Care | YES | NO | NA | Care Plan/Documentation | YES | NO | NA |
|---|---|---|---|---|---|---|---|
| 1. Satisfied with diet? | | | | I. Nursing/dietary orders re: | | | |
| 2. Patient knows diet Rx/reason? | | | | 1. Food preferences? | | | |
| 3. Patient knows food allowed? | | | | 2. Food allergies? | | | |
| 4. Patient assisted w/ meals? | | | | 3. Special diet/feeding needs ID? | | | |

## Appendix A *(continued)*

### F. Elimination

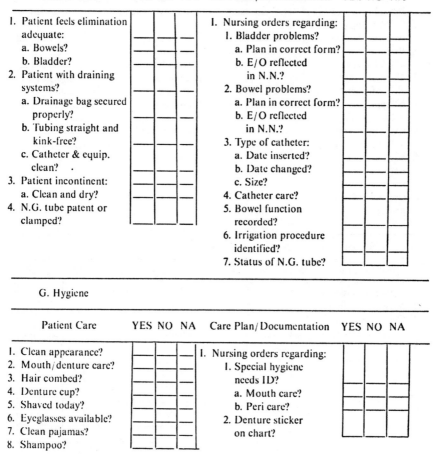

| Patient Care | YES | NO | NA | Care Plan/Documentation | YES | NO | NA |
|---|---|---|---|---|---|---|---|
| 1. Patient feels elimination adequate: | | | | 1. Nursing orders regarding: | | | |
|    a. Bowels? | | | |    1. Bladder problems? | | | |
|    b. Bladder? | | | |      a. Plan in correct form? | | | |
| 2. Patient with draining systems? | | | |      b. E/O reflected in N.N.? | | | |
|    a. Drainage bag secured properly? | | | |    2. Bowel problems? | | | |
|    b. Tubing straight and kink-free? | | | |      a. Plan in correct form? | | | |
|    c. Catheter & equip. clean? | | | |      b. E/O reflected in N.N.? | | | |
| 3. Patient incontinent: | | | |    3. Type of catheter: | | | |
|    a. Clean and dry? | | | |      a. Date inserted? | | | |
| 4. N.G. tube patent or clamped? | | | |      b. Date changed? | | | |
| | | | |      c. Size? | | | |
| | | | |    4. Catheter care? | | | |
| | | | |    5. Bowel function recorded? | | | |
| | | | |    6. Irrigation procedure identified? | | | |
| | | | |    7. Status of N.G. tube? | | | |

### G. Hygiene

| Patient Care | YES | NO | NA | Care Plan/Documentation | YES | NO | NA |
|---|---|---|---|---|---|---|---|
| 1. Clean appearance? | | | | 1. Nursing orders regarding: | | | |
| 2. Mouth/denture care? | | | |    1. Special hygiene needs ID? | | | |
| 3. Hair combed? | | | |      a. Mouth care? | | | |
| 4. Denture cup? | | | |      b. Peri care? | | | |
| 5. Shaved today? | | | |    2. Denture sticker on chart? | | | |
| 6. Eyeglasses available? | | | | | | | |
| 7. Clean pajamas? | | | | | | | |
| 8. Shampoo? | | | | | | | |

### H. Physical Comfort – Environment and Nursing Measures

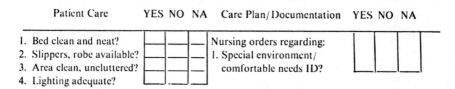

| Patient Care | YES | NO | NA | Care Plan/Documentation | YES | NO | NA |
|---|---|---|---|---|---|---|---|
| 1. Bed clean and neat? | | | | Nursing orders regarding: | | | |
| 2. Slippers, robe available? | | | | 1. Special environment/ comfortable needs ID? | | | |
| 3. Area clean, uncluttered? | | | | | | | |
| 4. Lighting adequate? | | | | | | | |

## Appendix A *(continued)*

| Patient Care | YES | NO | NA | Care Plan/Documentation | YES | NO | NA |
|---|---|---|---|---|---|---|---|
| 5. Special comfort measures: | | | | | | | |
| a. Blankets? | | | | | | | |
| b. Pillows? | | | | | | | |
| c. Drapes pulled? | | | | | | | |
| 6. Urinal available and clean? | | | | | | | |
| 7. Water glass clean? | | | | | | | |
| 8. Fresh water available? | | | | | | | |

### I. Rest and Sleep

| Patient Care | YES | NO | NA | Care Plan/Documentation | YES | NO | NA |
|---|---|---|---|---|---|---|---|
| 1. Patient sleeps at night? | | | | Nursing orders regarding: | | | |
| 2. Patient rests during the day? | | | | 1. Spec'l noc sleep needs ID? | | | |
| 3. Noise in the area? | | | | 2. Special rest needs ID? | | | |

### J. Safety

| Patient Care | YES | NO | NA | Care Plan/Documentation | YES | NO | NA |
|---|---|---|---|---|---|---|---|
| 1. Call light available? | | | | Nursing orders regarding: | | | |
| 2. Pt. knows how to use call light? | | | | 1. Patient in restraints/ posey? | | | |
| 3. Pt. knows how to use emergency signal? | | | | 2. Patient assistance when out of bed? | | | |
| 4. Side rails up? Positioned correctly? | | | | 3. Nursing orders for: | | | |
| 5. Bed in low position? | | | | a. Convulsion? | | | |
| 6. Radiation precautions? | | | | b. Radiation? | | | |
| 7. Floor dry, uncluttered? | | | | c. Isolation? | | | |
| 8. Isolation precautions observed? | | | | d. Oxygen? | | | |
| 9. Call light answered promptly? | | | | e. Allergies: | | | |
| | | | | Chart? | | | |
| 10. Preventing measure for falls? | | | | C.P.? | | | |
| a. Padded side rails? | | | | f. Falls? | | | |
| b. Restraints? | | | | g. Orient time & place? | | | |
| c. Sitter? | | | | 4. V/S charted BID? | | | |
| 11. Medications: | | | | | | | |
| a. Nurse watches when taken? | | | | | | | |
| b. At bedside? | | | | | | | |
| 12. Pt. band (allergies)? | | | | | | | |
| 13. $O_2$ in use (sign)? | | | | | | | |

**Appendix A** *(continued)*

## II. PSYCHO-SOCIAL NEEDS
A. Sense of Security

| Patient Care | YES | NO | NA | Care Plan/Documentation | YES | NO | NA |
|---|---|---|---|---|---|---|---|
| 1. Can the patient identify his or her nurse? | | | | I. Emotional status identified (on adm. form)? | | | |
| 2. Is there opportunity for patient to discuss fears and anxieties? | | | | II. Problem identified? | | | |
| 3. Patient's questions answered? | | | | III. Nursing orders? | | | |
| 4. Patient told about activities and procedures? | | | | IV. Plan in current form? | | | |
| 5. Pt. has confidence in nurses caring for him or her? | | | | V. E/O reflected in N. Notes? | | | |
| 6. Patient feels bored? | | | | | | | |
| 7. Patient feels lonely? | | | | | | | |
| 8. Patient depressed or anxious? | | | | | | | |
| 9. Patient feels privacy is being maintained? | | | | | | | |
| 10. Communication method established? | | | | | | | |
| 11. Religious needs being met? | | | | | | | |

## Appendix A *(continued)*

---

### III. TEACHING NEEDS

---

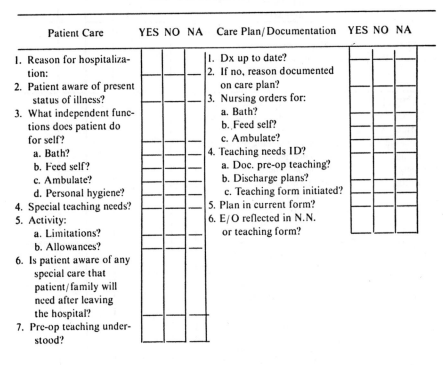

| Patient Care | YES | NO | NA | Care Plan/Documentation | YES | NO | NA |
|---|---|---|---|---|---|---|---|
| 1. Reason for hospitalization: | | | | 1. Dx up to date? | | | |
| 2. Patient aware of present status of illness? | | | | 2. If no, reason documented on care plan? | | | |
| 3. What independent functions does patient do for self? | | | | 3. Nursing orders for: | | | |
| a. Bath? | | | | a. Bath? | | | |
| b. Feed self? | | | | b. Feed self? | | | |
| c. Ambulate? | | | | c. Ambulate? | | | |
| d. Personal hygiene? | | | | 4. Teaching needs ID? | | | |
| 4. Special teaching needs? | | | | a. Doc. pre-op teaching? | | | |
| 5. Activity: | | | | b. Discharge plans? | | | |
| a. Limitations? | | | | c. Teaching form initiated? | | | |
| b. Allowances? | | | | 5. Plan in current form? | | | |
| 6. Is patient aware of any special care that patient/family will need after leaving the hospital? | | | | 6. E/O reflected in N.N. or teaching form? | | | |
| 7. Pre-op teaching understood? | | | | | | | |

---

### IV. HOSPITAL SAFETY

---

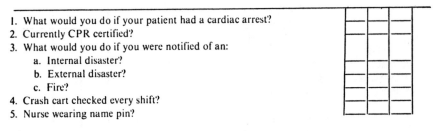

| | YES | NO | NA |
|---|---|---|---|
| 1. What would you do if your patient had a cardiac arrest? | | | |
| 2. Currently CPR certified? | | | |
| 3. What would you do if you were notified of an: | | | |
| a. Internal disaster? | | | |
| b. External disaster? | | | |
| c. Fire? | | | |
| 4. Crash cart checked every shift? | | | |
| 5. Nurse wearing name pin? | | | |

---

# Appendix B.  Guidelines for Integrating Nursing Process into Practice

| ACTIVITY | COMPONENTS | WK 1 | WK 2 | WK 3 | WK 4 | 3rd Mo. | Date & Init. Comp. |
|---|---|---|---|---|---|---|---|
| ASSESSMENT | 1. Admit patients to hospital following admission | | | X | | | |
| | 2. Document assessment data in chart and MIS | | | X | | | |
| NURSING CARE PLANNING | 1. Update nursing care plans in MIS as changes occur | | | X | | | |
| | 2. Formulate nursing care plans in MIS on assigned patients using the Mayer Model | | | | | X | |
| PATIENT TEACHING (with use of discharge teaching progress records) | 1. Identify teaching needs for assigned patients (standard or individualized) | | | X | | | |
| | 2. Develop teaching plans for assigned patients | | | | X | | |
| | 3. Implement teaching plans for assigned patients | | | | X | | |
| | 4. Evaluate each patient contact for learning achieved | | | | X | | |
| | 5. Document each patient teaching contact | | | | X | | |
| EVALUATION | 1. Ongoing evaluation of patient's response to care given | | | X | | | |
| ORGANIZA- TIONAL SKILLS | 1. Complete clinical unit skills inventory and update periodically | X | | | | | |
| | 2. Develop an individual system for collecting all pertinent information on assigned patients | | X | | | | |
| | 3. Begin administering direct nursing care to one acute and one intermediate patient | | X | | | | |
| | 4. Increase patient load to usual patient assignment for shift and clinical unit | | | X | | | |
| MIS ACTIVITIES Admission MD Orders Nursing Activities IV's/Blood OR— Transfer— Incident report Discharge/ expire | 1. Complete Learning Center MIS Modules assigned by instructor | X | | | | | |
| | 2. Practice MIS activities with preceptor or secretary coaching | | X | | | | |
| | 3. Perform MIS activities appropriate for patient care assignment | | | X | | | |

*Note:* For orientation of experienced RNs. Keep this with your skills inventory in your unit folder.

**Appendix C.    El Camino Hospital Flyer**

2500 GRANT ROAD • MOUNTAIN VIEW, CALIFORNIA 94042 • (415) 968-8111

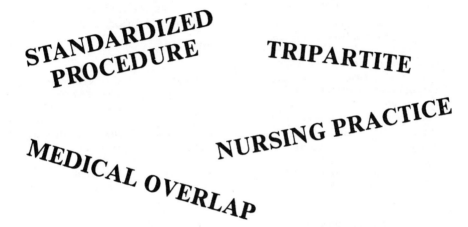

# *REMEMBER THESE TERMS?*

REMEMBER THESE TERMS?

El Camino Hospital Nurse Practice Committee will be discussing and deciding an important Nursing Practice issue dealing with management of the diabetic patient at El Camino.

All interested staff including diabetic resource members are invited to come to the next Nurse Practice Committee meeting on Thursday, February 19 at 3:30 in dining room "A."

## THIS IS A CHANCE
## FOR YOU TO DETERMINE
## NURSING PRACTICE AT EL CAMINO

*OPERATED BY EL CAMINO HOSPITAL DISTRICT*

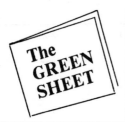

# NURSING SERVICE UPDATE

JANUARY 15, 1981
EL CAMINO HOSPITAL

## COMMITTEE REPORTS HIGHLIGHTS

*The new Executive Advisory Committee Members have decided on the theme "Closing The Gap" for their project. Their goal is to facilitate communications between all Nursing Staff through fun, socializing, and programs. Committee members are:*

| | |
|---|---|
| *Mary, CCU* | *Joy, ICU* |
| *Joyce* | *Rose, Nursery* |
| *Kathy, ER* | *Gerri, 6 West* |
| *Lynette, L&D* | *Janet* |
| *Vivian, 5 West* | *Veronica, 2W* |
| *Naomi, 2 North* | |

## INTERDEPARTMENTAL BULLETINS

AS OF JULY IST, TO PROVIDE A MORE EFFECTIVE CODE CPR TEAM THE ASSIGNMENTS AND TEAM MEMBERS HAVE BEEN REVISED AS FOLLOWS:

1. CCU –LEADER
2. TCU –MEDICATIONS
3. RT -RESPIRATORY SUPPORT
4. PATIENT'S OWN NURSE – MASSAGE
5. MSO ASSIGNED NURSE – RECORDER

WELCOME TCU! STAFF AND PA-TIENTS ALIKE APPRECIATE YOUR SUPPORT IN THIS EFFORT. YOUR BACKGROUND AND EXPERIENCE WITH THE CODE CPR PROTOCOL MEDS WILL ADD MUCH TO OUR RESUSCITATION EFFORTS. TO SUP-PORT THE CRITICAL-CARE UNITS DURING CODE CPR'S, MSO WILL SEND BACKUP STAFF TO TCU AND CCU.

## WEEKLY CALENDAR
(January 19–January 23, 1981)

MONDAY:
1/19

| | |
|---|---|
| TUESDAY:<br>1/20 | Exec. Committee<br>8:00 – 9:30 AM<br>Dining Room "C" |
| WEDNESDAY:<br>1/21 | Night Staff/Human<br>Support<br>Coffee and<br>Conversation<br>7:45 AM<br>Dining Room "E" |
| | Physical Assessment<br>Series<br>Chest Exam –Part<br>II<br>3rd Floor Solarium<br>See listing on unit<br>for times. |
| | Ostomy Resource<br>Committee<br>3:30 PM<br>Dining Room "D" |
| THURSDAY:<br>1/22 | |
| FRIDAY:<br>1/23 | Nursing Care<br>Planning<br>9:15AM–1:15 PM<br>Dining Room "A" |

A BIG THANKS TO ALL PERSONNEL THAT FLOATED TO 2N DURING THE HOLIDAYS!

2N STAFF

## INTERDEPARTMENTAL BULLETINS CONTINUED

WELCOME to Conrad, our new Patient Transporter, who will be working evenings. After orienting with Fidel, he will start working on the 2:00 PM - 8:00PM Shift, Monday, Jan. 19, 1980.

On Jan. 19th, we will be back to our regular coverage of 7:30AM - 8:00PM, Mon. through Fri.; & 7:30 11:30AM, Saturday. Thank you for your patience the past month.

## AVAILABLE IN CENTRAL SERVICE: HOLLISTER STERILE DRAINAGE SYSTEM
5cm size AND 8cm size.

## ATTENTION: NEW COMMITTEE

A task force met to establish a new committee called Nursing Care Review Committee. This committee will be responsible for reviewing incidents in nursing that require remedial action to maintain high quality care and establish ongoing educational programs. The selection process consists of the following criteria:

1. Maintain high degree of confidentiality.
2. Tenure at El Camino Hospital a minimum of 2 years.
3. Have served or are serving on Nurse Practice or Nursing Care Planning.
4. Demonstrate high quality nursing skills.
5. Willing to serve for a minimum of 1 year with 90% attendance.
6. Committed to process and meetings.

Please submit application in writing to Quality Assurance Coordinators. Existing task force will review applications and select committee members. Any questions, please contact Nancy or Virginia. Criteria for selection is negotiable.

## EDUCATION PROGRAMS. FOR YOUR PATIENTS NOW SHOWING ON FREE T.V.

All ECH patients and their families can now view 14 different health-related educational programs on FREE Channel 13 of their bedside TV. The special TV guide listing these programs and their scheduled viewing times is available on all nursing units from unit clerk. This guide should be given to each new ECH patient by the nurse responsible for admitting the patient. The success of this new service depends on your active promotion of the programs to patients. We encourage you to become familiar with the content and viewing times of programs appropriate to your patients.

*PRECEPTORS! Watch for announcement of preceptor update on the forthcoming changes in orientation necessitated by the addition of 1 day "General Hospital". Plan to come and see what's happening—and get your questions answered.*

## INTERDEPARTMENTAL BULLETINS STAFF NURSE III TASK FORCE

A group of expert El Camino Hospital nurses has been selected to participate in a Task Force to describe Staff Nurse III performance. The group will (1) develop criteria for Staff Nurse III eligibility; (2) propose methods for implementation beginning July 1, 1981; and (3) propose methods for ongoing validation of Staff Nurse III Practice. The Task Force will hold its first meeting Monday, February 9th. We have retained the consultation services of Ruth, R.N., M.S., who is the associate director of the AMICAE project, USF, to assist us with this endeavor. Ann will be chairing the Task Force and the group members include Pam, 2E; Danielle, 5W; Michelle, 6W; Shirley, L&D; Denise, Peds; Stephanie, TCU; Linda, R.R.; Judy, O.R.; Louise, AKU; Kay, Psych; Donnie, ER; Nancy, Staff Development; Elaine, Nursing Administration.

## CONGRATULATIONS

Congratulations to Jan on being selected as Head Nurse for 6 West. Jan is currently Acting Head Nurse on 2 East and will move into her new role on 6 West in the very near future. Once Jan is oriented Elaine, current 6 West Head Nurse will move to her new job as Nursing Coordinator.

## ECH CURRENT CAREER OPPORTUNITIES

Head Nurse position open on 6E, a dynamic medical primary nursing unit. Interested nurses with previous leadership experience and a minimum of 2 years' clinical experience in medical nursing, please contact Patti, Ext. 44543, for further details. B.S. in Nursing preferred.

## CRITICAL-CARE FLOAT

Requires strong Critical-Care background and hemodymanic monitoring skills. Would include floating to Cardiac Cath Lab. Days, Monday thru Friday. Make application to Mary, CCU, or June, Cardiac Cath Lab.

## FIRST-AID INSTRUCTOR

A job-enrichment opportunity will be available for a First-Aid Instructor beginning January, 1981. This individual will be responsible for conducting an 8-hour first-aid course. Classes will be taught through the LifeCheck Program in local industry on a limited basis. Classes will be scheduled as the program grows. Requirements for the position: (1) certified first-aid instructor; (2) previous first-aid teaching experience; (3) flexibility to increase hours as the program grows; and (4) availability during the hours 8-5 for training sessions. For more information call M., Ext. 44551 or 44619. Deadline: January 26, 1981.

## INFECTION-CONTROL COORDINATOR

Position opportunity available for an RN who has had prior experience as an Infection-Control Nurse with responsibility for the total infection-control program in a comparable acute hospital setting. BSN or MSN preferred. Full-time position. For details call Patti, RN Coord. Nurse Recruitment. Ext. 4454.

### MSO

|  |  |
|---|---|
| 3 West -Surgical Mary, HN | 2 RNs 3/5 PT 7 - 1 RN PD 7 3 every other weekend. 1 RN 4/5 PT 3-11 1 RN PD -1/5-2/5 11-7 |
| 6 West -Medical Elaine, HN | Head Nurse 1 RN FT 3-11 |
| 6 East -Medical Gladys, HN | 1 AHN FT 11-7 1 RN 4/5-FT 3-11 CUS 3/5 PT 3-11 |
| MSO Floats apply to Corrine, HN | 1 RN FT 7-3 1 RN 4/5 PT 3-11 2 RNs FT 11-7 |

### MCH

|  |  |
|---|---|
| L&D Carolyn, HN | 1 RN UNSC PD 11-7 |
| Pediatrics Sherryn, HN | 1 NA 2/5-3/5 3-1 |

### CRITICAL CARE

|  |  |
|---|---|
| TCU Pat, HN | 1 RN PT 3-11 1 RN PT 11-7 1 RN FT 11-7 |
| ICU Sally, HN | 1 AHN FT 11-7 |
| CCU Mary, HN | RN's FT/PT/PD 11 $10^0$ shift -4 days |
| Critical Care Floats apply to Pat, HN | RN's FT/PT/PD 11-7 |
| AKU Marilyn, HN | RN's FT/PT 7-3 RN's FT/PT 3-11 |

## Appendix E.   New Employee Progress Evaluation

## NEW EMPLOYEE PROGRESS EVALUATION

☐ Days
☐ Evenings
☐ Nights

Orientee's Names: _____ Date: _____
Preceptor's Name: _____ Unit: _____

Strengths                                  Areas to Improve

Behavioral Objectives (to meet areas needing improvement):            Time Frame:

SIGNATURES

New Employee: _____

Preceptor: _____

H.N./A.H.N.: _____

This form is to be completed in duplicate. One copy is to be kept in the employee's professional profile, and one copy forwarded to the staff development instructor. It should be completed by the preceptor and new employee jointly. One form is to be completed at the end of day orientation and another at the end of shift orientation.

## Appendix F.    Hospital Organizational Chart

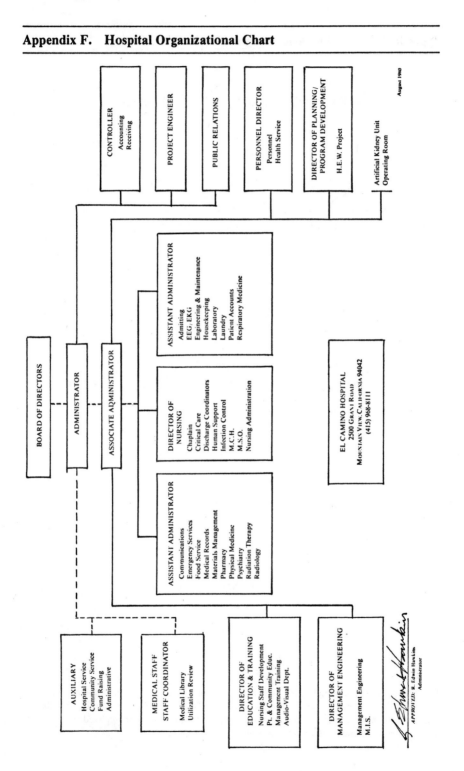

August 1980

BOARD OF DIRECTORS

ADMINISTRATOR

ASSOCIATE ADMINISTRATOR

CONTROLLER
Accounting
Receiving

PROJECT ENGINEER

PUBLIC RELATIONS

PERSONNEL DIRECTOR
Personnel
Health Service

DIRECTOR OF PLANNING/
PROGRAM DEVELOPMENT
H.E.W. Project

Artificial Kidney Unit
Operating Room

ASSISTANT ADMINISTRATOR
Admitting
EEG/EKG
Engineering & Maintenance
Housekeeping
Laboratory
Laundry
Patient Accounts
Respiratory Medicine

DIRECTOR OF
NURSING
Chaplain
Critical Care
Discharge Coordinators
Human Support
Infection Control
M.C.H.
M.S.O.
Nursing Administration

ASSISTANT ADMINISTRATOR
Communications
Emergency Services
Food Service
Medical Records
Materials Management
Pharmacy
Physical Medicine
Psychiatry
Radiation Therapy
Radiology

EL CAMINO HOSPITAL
2500 GRANT ROAD
MOUNTAIN VIEW, CALIFORNIA 94042
(415) 968-8111

AUXILIARY
Hospital Service
Community Service
Fund Raising
Administrative

MEDICAL STAFF
STAFF COORDINATOR
Medical Library
Utilization Review

DIRECTOR OF
EDUCATION & TRAINING
Nursing Staff Development
Pt. & Community Educ.
Management Training
Audio-Visual Dept.

DIRECTOR OF
MANAGEMENT ENGINEERING
Management Engineering
M.I.S.

*APPROVED:* R. Edwin Hawkins
Administrator

**Appendix G.**

# NURSING SERVICE

# ANNUAL REPORT 1980

## Compiled by Suzanne Schauwecker

# ANNUAL REPORT
# Contents

*Nursing Service Organization*

El Camino Hospital's Decentralized Nursing Structure

*Organizational Charts*

*Goals and Achievements*

Director of Nursing Services Report

*Education and Training Support Review*

Education and Training Director's Report
Management Training/Organization Development (MOD) Instructor's Report
General Education Instructor's Report
Health Education Service Report
Nursing Education Instructors' Report
MSO Complex Instructors' Report
MCH Complex Instructors' Report
Critical-Care Complex Instructors' Report

*Nursing Coordinator Review*

Financing and Staffing Coordinator's Report
Nurse Recruitment and Employee Relations Coordinator's Report
Interdepartment Nursing Liaison Coordinator's Report
Quality Assurance Coordinator's Report
Nursing Audit Coordinator's Report
Report of the Nursing Coordinators, 3 – 11 Shift
Report of the Nursing Coordinators, 11 – 7 Shift
Infection Control Coordinator's Report
Discharge Planning Coordinators' Report

*Nursing Unit Review*

Emergency Department Head Nurse's Report
Intensive Care Unit Head Nurse's Report
Cardiac Care Unit Head Nurse's Report
Transitional Care Unit Head Nurse's Report
Labor and Delivery Head Nurse's Report
Nursery Head Nurse's Report
Maternity.Head Nurse's Report
Pediatrics Head Nurse's Report
2-North (Surgical) Head Nurse's Report
2-West (Surgical) Head Nurse's Report
2-East (Surgical) Head Nurse's Report
5-West (Surgical) Head Nurse's Report
5-East (Orthopedic) Head Nurse's Report
6-West (Medical) Head Nurse's Report
6-East (Medical) Head Nurse's Report

*Committee and Task Force Review*

CPR Committee Chairperson's Report
Diabetic Resource Committee Chairperson's Report
MIS Committee Chairperson's Report
Nurse Practice Committee Chairperson's Report
Nursing Care Planning Committee Chairperson's Report
Nursing Care Review Committee's Report
Ostomy Resource Committee Chairperson's Report
Product Evaluation Committee's Report
Reach-to-Recovery Resource Committee Chairperson's Report

**Exhibit 2–1.   Line Staff Relationship
of DNS to Nursing Unit Staff**

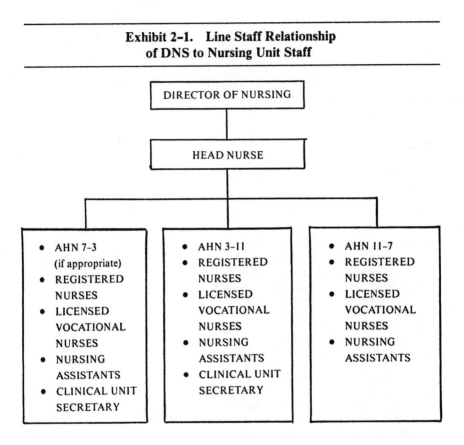

**Exhibit 2–2.   Line and Support Staff
Nursing Service Organization**

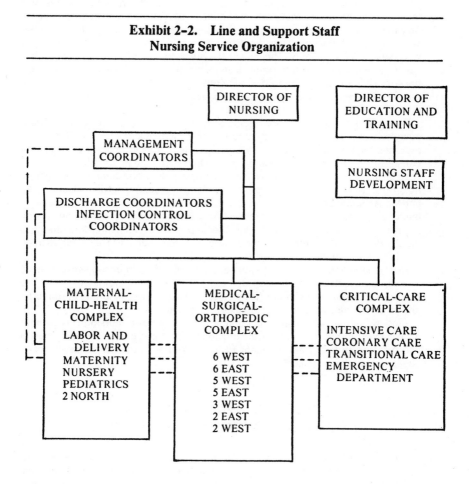

## EL CAMINO HOSPITAL'S
## DECENTRALIZED NURSING STRUCTURE

It is the belief of the El Camino Hospital nursing service that patient care is enhanced when accountability for decision and actions is vested in the professionals closest to the patients. This means that each individual nurse realizes a high degree of auton-omy in making decisions for the patient. In this setting the responsible nurse inter-acts directly with the physician, dietitian, pharmacist, etc., in planning care for and with the patient and family. This allows the nurse to maintain an assertive profes-sional and satisfying role while maximizing her education and skills. This is possible because each nursing unit is a discrete entity responsible for its organization and patient care milieu. There is a direct line of accountability between the director of nursing and the head nurse of each unit.

The various nursing units are organized into three "complex" groupings. These complexes are the Medical-Surgical-Orthopedic Complex, the Critical Care Com-plex, and the Maternal Child Health Complex. Head nurses meet regularly in their complexes to problem solve, analyze issues, and exchange information.

To facilitate participative management decision making and communication flow, nursing service has two management committees, Executive Advisory Committee, and Management Council. The Executive Advisory Committee is a nursing manage-ment committee comprised of representatives from all job categories within nursing service, including all three shifts. Membership rotates every three months. This group meets at least monthly with the director of nursing service to review and screen issues for the Management Council.

The Management Council is comprised of the director of nursing services, head nurses, representatives from staff development and the coordinator group. The council meets monthly to analyze problems, make recommendations to the director, and reach consensus on nursing policies and issues.

Each individual staff nurse, each unit, and the director of nursing service have access to resources that collectively provide support and guidance. This group of coordinators and staff development instructors offers expertise in patient care, education, and management.

## GOALS AND ACHIEVEMENTS
## Director of Nursing Service's Report

Amidst soaring health-care costs, a growing nurse shortage, and an overall escalat-ing inflationary rate, we in nursing have felt "tugs" of a stronger and somewhat different nature this year. In reality our client, the patient, has also been affected directly or indirectly by all these factors. Yet our goal in nursing has remained that of providing quality nursing care to our patients while maintaining emphasis on cost containment and staff satisfaction.

This fiscal year, July 1979 to July 1980, our overall hospital budget was 41.2 million dollars. Of that budget, total Nursing Service claimed 17.5 million. Nursing Service as a single division had, and still has, the highest component of the work force. Thus nursing labor alone accounted for 36.8% of the total hospital wage packet.

To illustrate the degree of budget responsibility at the nursing unit level, each head nurse, on the average, managed a million-dollar budget. This million-dollar budget reflects both direct costs (wages, benefits, supplies, etc.), and indirect costs (overhead, depreciation). On the nursing unit level, 50% of the cost was labor.

A labor productivity goal of .963 was set by total Nursing Service this year. Our actual achievement was that of .973—an achievement of .01 above goal. As a means of illustrating the dollar impact in relationship to labor productivity achievement or nonachievement, we might point out that for Nursing Service each productivity point variance from goal was worth, on the average, $3448 per pay period.

Nursing's achievement in labor productivity is an indicator not only of responsible management but of a cost containment effort as well. Besides careful labor productivity monitoring, nursing looks at other means of cost containment, including supplies, new products, and services evaluation.

Prior to budget preparation, nursing collects data while studying El Camino Hospital patient trends. The following were major factors influencing budget redistribution for the '79-'80 nursing unit budgets: (1) overall rise in patient acuity level; (2) change in major/minor surgery mix with a documented increase in the major mix; (3) increase in number of patients age 65 and above; (4) the average length of patient stay stable at 5.3 days; (5) change in the GYN patient mix; and (6) the number of patients on hyperalimentation on designated units. With data base, these factors provided rationale for negotiating change in labor standards for given nursing units.

In the yearly budgeting process, the head nurse negotiates with the director of nursing service the unit patient care productivity goal. During the year, the head nurse alone and with the director of nursing service reviews and analyzes actual goal achievement and impacts affecting that achievement. This total process enhances future budget planning.

The concern for productivity monitoring and cost containment is possible because nursing holds paramount the delivery of quality care to all our patients. In order to evaluate our success in providing quality care, we currently utilize three measurement systems:

*1. Concurrent patient care audit system.* This system is perhaps the most relevant for us in nursing because it occurs while the patient is in the hospital. Due to its timeliness, we have an opportunity to make immediate changes/improvements in the patient's care if it is deemed necessary.

Concurrent audits are conducted on all nursing units at least three times a year. A minimum of four nursing units are audited each month. The nursing units are scheduled for audit on a random basis in order to avoid purposeful skewing of the data collected.

The actual process as it occurs on the nursing unit is as follows: Approximately 25% of the unit patient census, or seven to eight patients on the average nursing unit, are randomly selected by a nursing coordinator; the nursing coordinator interviews each of the patients selected; she compares the information about the patient with the nursing care plan and the nurses' notes, and then she interviews the nursing care for the patient. Six different parameters of care are measured for each patient, with three parameters falling under the patient care component and three under the care planning component. The three parameters measured in each component are (1) physical, (2) psychosocial, and (3) therapeutic/rehabilitative care needs.

Scores from the seven or eight patient care audits are then compiled and a unit score is developed. The results of the audit are reviewed with the nursing unit staff within 24–48 hours when possible.

In the last year the concurrent audit scores compiled for total nursing revealed an attainment of an overall score of 92%, with a score of 98% in the patient care component and an 89% in the care planning component. Our goal had been to reach a score of 90% or above in each parameter of care measured. Thus, our focus now is to raise the care planning component score while maintaining our achievement in the patient care component.

*2. Retrospective chart reviews or audits.* This year retrospective audits have been conducted on the following: intraocular lens implant, Emergency Room, episodic depressive disorder, bunion surgery, pacemaker, and, intraoperative management of general, spinal and epiderial anesthesia.

Criteria for the retrospective nursing audits are set up by nurse clinicians and the nursing audit and quality assurance coordinators. Any nursing deficiencies found on a retrospective audit are communicated to the appropriate head nurse. She, with the help of the quality assurance coordinator, develops a remedial action plan. The head nurse submits this plan to the director of nursing service and quality assurance coordinator. The head nurse shares the audit information and the remedial action plan with her staff. Implementation of the plan then occurs. To check the effectiveness of the remedial action plan, retrospective audits are again conducted on patient the remedial action plan implementation.

*3. Post-discharge questionnaires.* The patient is asked to respond to questions specific to different aspects of his/her care with ample space allotted for comments. The patient may remain anonymous if he/she chooses. Feedback gathered in this manner gives nursing another means whereby we can evaluate our services, identify general or specific problems, or gain reassurance that our care is perceived by the patient as being positive and meeting his/her needs.

This year, 1837 questionnaires were sent to patients post discharge. Of these, 1054 were returned (a 57% return). The majority of responses to the nursing care aspects were most positive. An overall score of 94% was achieved.

Results of the questionnaires were then shared with the head nurse of those nursing units whose patients had been polled. She in turn shared this information with her staff. The nursing unit then made adjustments to their care delivery if and as appropriate.

Highly interrelated to achievement in productivity, cost containment, and quality patient care is staff retention (or conversely, staff turnover). Our nursing unit average turnover rate for 1980 was 14%. This shows a decrease of 5.7% from the previous year.

In comparison to most hospitals in the area, our turnover rate is considered on the low side. However, we have experienced increasing difficulty in recruiting RNs to fill vacated and new positions. These new positions are created because of the increasing acuity of our patients, which results in the need for more RNs, coupled with the desire of many nurses to reduce the number of hours or days they work each week.

In keeping with our goal to have adequate numbers of qualified nurses providing care to our patients, we have implemented a critical-care nursing course in conjunction with De Anza College. To date we have hired 27 nurses with no prior critical-care nursing experience and have educated them to work in our critical care units. We also increased the number of new nursing graduates that we employ, a total of 27 were hired last year. We have been delighted with the ease with which they have made the transition from student to professional nurse. We attribute much of the success of the new graduate and other employee orientation programs to our highly skilled nurse preceptors.

A completely new endeavor this year was our participation with Stanford Hospital, Veterans Hospital, and De Anza College to "refresh" nurses in order that they could confidently reenter the nursing job market. Our nursing staff on the 3–11 shift served as preceptors and mentors for a group of six women who were completing the clinical component of the refresher program. Three of the six are now permanent members of our staff.

One of the problems a busy and decentralized organization such as ours experiences is the difficulty of keeping everyone informed about the many exciting and creative things our staff is accomplishing. Providing an opportunity where staff could meet new colleagues, renew old friendships, and get an "update" was deemed important. Therefore this fall we had our first annual party and information exchange. Over 200 of the nursing staff attended the event.

Overall, this year has been a year of progress and growth for us. Nursing's positive achievement of goals set has been attained through the expertise, the hard work, and the commitment of all the nursing staff.

# EDUCATION AND TRAINING SUPPORT REVIEW

## EDUCATION AND TRAINING DIRECTOR'S REPORT

The nursing department is the largest client of education and training services in the hospital. This is readily understandable when one considers that the product of the hospital industry is patient care and that patients spend the majority of their time in the hospital being ministered to by nursing department personnel. Education and training support to the nursing department is broad ranged. It includes the knowledge and skill-building programming of orientation, technical skill training, continuing education, and management development. It also includes staff support for projects, task forces, and committee work.

A large component of education and training support to the nursing department is in the form of internal consultation in which lone managers are assisted with analyzing the work environment, exploring alternative actions, choosing courses of action and evaluating results. Health education service consults with nursing department personnel on patient-education programs and also provides direct patient-education services as prescribed.

Modern approaches to staff development have been used in the nursing department, e.g., the independent self-paced learning model, learning center, and Core Curriculum. Job variety and job enrichment opportunities have been provided through such activities as preceptorship, development of resource nurse groups and train-the-trainer activities. The education and training department and the nursing departments have a long history of successful enterprises that have resulted in improved patient care services and enhanced employee development.

## MANAGEMENT TRAINING/ORGANIZATION DEVELOPMENT (MOD) INSTRUCTOR'S REPORT

My major achievements this year have been:

- Head nurses and assistant head nurses continue to participate in the hospital's basic and continuing education MOD programs.
    1. *Basic* —Leadership, Communications, Job Clarification, Coaching & Performance Review, Time Management, Personnel Aspects of Supervision, Stress Management, Creative Problem Solving, Management Cycle.
    2. *Continuing Education*—Speed Reading, Coaching for Improved Job Performance.
    3. *Group Facilitation*—Nursing department has availed itself of group facilitation consultation.

My major goals for the coming year are:

- MOD programs that will have positive impact for nursing service are:
    1. *Management Cycle*—Increased coordination of Nursing Unit/Department goals with overall hospital goals.
    2. *Internal Consultation*—Improved consultation process between line managers and staff support persons.
    3. *Basic and C.E. MOD*—Increased management skills of HNs and AHNs through participation in scheduled MOD programs.

## GENERAL EDUCATION INSTRUCTOR'S REPORT

The General Educator provides Education & Training staff support to all hospital departments and develops generic educational programs that cross two or more department lines.

My major achievements this year have been:

- *Back Care Program*—a training-the-trainers model was used to prepare department and unit representatives for training their work group in 30-minute sessions in techniques of safe lifting. This program is directed at increasing the safety and well-being of hospital employees and decreasing hospital costs related to employee injuries.
- *Dealing with Combative Patients*—In a one-day workshop, Emergency and Psychiatry employees and nursing employees from selective, high-risk areas were taught safe and effective techniques for dealing with combative patients. Eight of those participants were selected for an intense five-day train-the-trainer program in which they learned how to teach future programs in this content area.
- *General Hospital Orientation*—All new employees spend first day of employment in general hospital orientation including meeting hospital administrator and learning about safety, employee benefits, stress management and employees' association. Nurses participate in this and then go to nursing orientation next day.

My major goals for the coming year are:

- Future programs that will include participation from the nursing department are:
    1. Dealing with Combative Patients (primarily E.R., Med-Surg., Psychiatry)
    2. First Contact Communications
    3. Safety Month (early 1981)

## HEALTH EDUCATION SERVICE REPORT

The Health Education Service was established in January, 1976, to promote, implement, and evaluate programs designed to help individuals adopt and maintain healthy practices and lifestyles. Staff in the service are available as resources to any nurse interested in developing programs/materials for patient teaching. We have current books, journals, and teaching materials in our office.

Program summary:

- Stress Management, Physical Fitness and Nutrition workshops were offered to five electronic industries in Santa Clara County, reaching 128 employees.
- In February, 1980, health-hazard appraisal was implemented in three local industries, reaching 114 individuals in this first five-month period.
- An average of 20 patients per month have been seen in the audiovisual Health Education Center with a referring base of 70 physicians.
- El Camino's Health Education Service was the model community outreach program showcased at the Third National Symposium on Patient Education in Baltimore, March 1980.
- Our community outreach efforts have resulted in our cosponsoring (1) an adolescent program with Mountain View/Los Altos Adult Education and (2) two health forums with the De Anza short-course program. In addition, we are advertising classes in each of their catalogues, reaching approximately 200,000 homes in our community.
- ECH employees now have the opportunity to register for any of our behavior-change workshops. To date, 58 employees have taken advantage of this opportunity.
- We have had direct contact with approximately 4,602 individuals in our hospital district during 1979-80.

## NURSING EDUCATION INSTRUCTORS' REPORTS

Nursing education instructors are responsible for jointly planning, developing, implementing, and evaluating generic programs that cross clinical complex lines and that meet knowledge/skill requirements in the most cost-effective manner possible.

The major achievements this year have been:

- *CPR* training has been updated and is provided during orientation and four times a year on all three shifts for recertification of nursing personnel. Auxilians have been trained as basic CPR instructors to assist in CPR training sessions. There is follow-up from CPR critiques and medication and CPR record review provided for nursing staff. In the last year, 467 nursing personnel have been certified and/or recertified.

- *Preceptor Program:* Between May 1979 and May 1980, two preceptor workshops were given and 56 nurses attended these workshops. Another preceptor workshop is scheduled for November 1980. Clinical follow-up for preceptors and new employees is provided. Orientation tools have been updated.
- *Physical assessment series* is available in the learning center for all nursing personnel. Classes are held four times monthly in one subject area in the hospital so that all nursing personnel can attend; 12 modules have been developed in various subject areas for this series.
- *Learning center* was moved to the first floor and condensed in size. Orientation to the learning center is provided for all new RNs and LVNs. Programs are added to the learning center frequently and the master list is updated twice a year. Instructors have shown the learning center to interested nurses from other facilities.
- *Hyperalimentation* program continues. Nurses on 2E, 5W, 6W, TCU, and ICU are being certified. In the past year, 26 nurses have been certified.
- *Patient Teaching:* Education and training staff worked with the diabetic, ostomy, and cardiac rehab resource nurses for updating and support of each program.
- *Shared educational services:* Ostomy series, pain, ACLS.

The major goals for the coming year are:

Major education and training goals that will have positive results for the nursing department are:

- Increasing clinical placement of students from both basic and refresher nursing programs to support nurse recruitment efforts.
- Continued and possibly increased utilization of community-college educational programming for both cost effectiveness and recruitment efforts.
- Increased challenge opportunities in core curriculum for validation of knowledge and skill and cost effectiveness.
- Exploration of computer-assisted instruction beginning with the content of MIS training.

## MSO COMPLEX INSTRUCTORS' REPORT

We are responsible for planning, developing, implementing, and evaluating educational programs and activities which promote individual development of MSO staff nurses. This is provided on a 24-hour basis.

The major accomplishments this year have been

- *Core curriculum* integrated into orientation process. HNs are encouraged to use Core Curriculum as a measurement for evaluation of staff.
- *Orientation* for Nursing Service was updated and reorganized. MIS modules and Orientation Tools were updated. Orientation Manual for each unit was provided and utilized during orientation. One hundred ninety-eight Nursing Service personnel have been oriented between September 1979–September 1980.
- *Learning center* programs have been purchased for Physical Assessment Series and CPR. The Master List has been updated.
- *Discharge teaching progress records* have been utilized by all MSO units. The

content was incorporated into the revised Patient Admission Interview Form.
- *Physical assessment series* was provided inhouse for all MSO units. One part of the series was presented every month on all three shifts. Attendance at each program is listed below:

| | |
|---|---:|
| Communication | 123 |
| The interview | 75 |
| The health history | 76 |
| Vital signs | 77 |
| Head & neck exam | 90 |
| Ear exam | 101 |
| Eye exam | 92 |
| Breast exam | 97 |
| Abdominal exam | In progress |

Lung exam, heart exam and neuro exam are in the learning center and will be presented in months to come.
- *Scheduled instructor clinical time* for all units weekly as clinical unit resource. Pediatrics is now a part of MSO staff development.
- *CPR medication nurse* (11-7) was developed for the unique CPR needs of 11-7 shift.
- *Continuous Ambulatory Peritoneal Dialysis (CAPD)* policies and procedures written. Training program was developed to assist 5W nurses in caring for inhouse CAPD patients.
- *Clinical resource* for HNs, coordinator, and staff nurse attending St. Mary's program. Time spent assisting in development of projects and implementation of studies. (CPR project, revision of policy manual, IV study, MIS module update.)
- *Consultant* to staff development instructors from other facilities on development of S.D. role, preceptor program, learning center, and computer training.
- *Management consultant* for HNs, AHNs, regarding personnel performance problems.
- *Refresher nurse program* through De Anza College was developed; needs assessment and training workshop provided. Refresher nurses will start clinical time in November 1980 with 3-11 MSO instructor as inhouse coordinator for this program.
- *Co-trainer for MOD sessions* regarding coaching, job clarification, and performance reviews.
- *CPR recertification* of all MSO nursing personnel through CPR marathons.

The major goals for the coming year are:

- *Hyperalimentation certification*—continue to certify RNs on 2E, 5W, 6W, ICU, TCU.
- *CPR*—100% of MSO nursing personnel will be recertified yearly.
- *Orientation/preceptor*—two preceptors per unit per shift will be prepared to actively function in that role.
- *Clinical resource*—MSO Instructors will be available on a weekly basis on each clinical unit on each shift and will be available as needed for clinical consultation.
- *Core curriculum*—foster use of core curriculum on each MSO unit.
- *Discharge teaching*—encourage utilization of discharge teaching tools.
- Revision of nursing care planning module.
- Feasibility of computer-assisted MIS training.
- Diabetic skills training workshop in Spring 1981
- Patient-teaching workshop, Spring 1981.

- Cancer resource nurse group will be established and ongoing.
- A study will be undertaken to look at potential revision of acuity systems.

## MCH COMPLEX INSTRUCTOR'S REPORT

Responsible for identifying real and potential learning needs of MCH Staff and for providing formal and informal programs and activities to meet these needs. Serves as clinical resource on all three shifts in Labor and Delivery, Nursery, and Maternity. Responsive to perinatal-oriented learning needs on the Pediatric Unit.

The major achievements this year have been:

*Cesarean section training*—Organized workshop to train six labor-and-delivery nurses to circulate for cesarean sections in the L&D suite.
*Core curriculum*—Organized a core curriculum task force for each of the four MCH units. These committees, composed of three preceptors and an instructor, each meet four hours/month for the purpose of developing a core curriculum for their respective units. Development of all four core curricula is scheduled to be completed by March 1981.
*Advanced newborn resuscitation training*—MCH instructor and nursery head nurse developed and now offer training in advanced newborn CPR four times/year. Content includes filmstrips and video tapes followed by practice sessions in use of bag and mask, cardiac compression, assistance with endotracheal intubation, and use of drugs. To date, 35 staff members from nursery, L&D, and maternity have completed the training program. This training will be offered to the pediatric nursing staff starting in November 1980.
*Breast-feeding conference*—A four hour conference on breast feeding and the nutritional aspects of breast milk was organized by MCH instructor and educator from the state-funded Santa Clara Perinatal Project. The program, given at El Camino Hospital in April 1980, had 25 attendees primarily composed of MCH nursing staff from El Camino Hospital. Video taped segments of the conference are available in the learning center and have been used extensively by the MCH staff.

The major goals for the coming year are:

*Modularization of cesarean section training*—MCH instructor is working with a staff nurse in L&D to develop a modularized program to train the L&D nursing staff to scrub and circulate for cesarean sections. Such a program will replace costly didactic workshops with self-paced, independent acquisition of theory followed by a precepted practicum. The extent to which this program is developed is dependent upon the somewhat tenuous notion that L&D will continue to expand its volume of surgical cases.
*Implementation of core curricula*—Upon completion of their development, the four MCH Core Curricula will be integrated into unit orientations and used as a source of educational support and performance standards for the existing staff.
*Computer-assisted care planning*—CACP is scheduled to be available to the three perinatal units in November 1980. Development of training program to facilitate this transition is currently in progress. The *Maternity Teaching Progress Record* will be implemented in conjunction with CACP.

## CRITICAL-CARE COMPLEX INSTRUCTORS' REPORT

The Critical Care instructors are responsible for providing special assistance and support to nurses in four critical-care units by identifying and providing formal and informal educational opportunities to meet assessed learning needs to promote professional growth and enhance delivery of quality patient care.

The major achievements this year have been:

- *Program development and implementation*
    1. Sixty-five new learning packages related to CC core curriculum
    2. Electrical safety modules for orientation
    3. Basic critical-care course (108° theory + self-paced instruction on competency model)
    4. Five-part emergency assessment course
    5. Three-level core curriculum for TCU
    6. CPR training project for ECH auxilians
    7. AKU—workshops for nursing leadership group on conflict management, coaching and development and workshops for RNs in respiratory physical assessment

- On-going courses, programs
    1. Five ACLS certification programs for CC RNs and ER physicians
    2. ACLS recertification programs (one at El Camino Hospital)
    3. Seventy-two Mock Code drill sessions for critical care RNs to maintain and improve CPR skills
    4. Twenty critical care RNs certified in chest assessment skills
    5. De Anza Community College
        -3 CCU Courses
        -2 Hemo dynamic monitoring courses
        -1 fluid & electrolyte course for refresher RNs

- *Consultation/resource*
    *Internal:*
    1. Precepted HN in B.A. program at St. Mary's
    2. Precepted SJS student in MPH program
    3. Precepted UC doctoral student in renal
    4. Weekly clinical unit resource activity
    *External:*
    1. Kaiser Hospital Administrator re: learning center
    2. Critical-care HN and educator from San Jose Hospital

The major goals for the coming year are:

Two new critical-care instructors are being oriented to the education and training functions and responsibilities in critical care.
- Complete critical-care core curriculum development
- Maintain the many critical-care programs and activities already in place

# NURSING COORDINATOR REVIEW

## FINANCE AND STAFFING COORDINATOR'S REPORT

Resource person to nursing service staff in areas of budget and staffing. Emphasis on the HN and AHN group. Develop systems which will promote efficiency, assist in coaching and development, provide training sessions, monitor performance, and effect a long-range planning mode/concept.

My major achievements this year have been:

- Oriented four new HNs to budget and staffing process.
- Oriented three management engineers to nursing service organization with focus on budgets and staffing.
- Developed teaching/training budget and staffing sessions for AHNs and staff nurses.
- Coaching/development HNs, AHNs and staff nurses in problem solving.
- Resource to NA, three staffing clerks and one secretary.
- Resource to some departments other than nursing for budget process.
- Coordinated budget workshop for all nursing units-increased numbers of partic- ipants in each session to include staff nurses and SD group
- Active participant in Forecasting Committee.
- Monitored performance of HNs, provided input to their evaluations in areas of budgets/staffing.
- Worked on specific projects, i.e., float policy development, L&D ABC program, opening/closing units, budget and staffing systems consultation.
- President of El Camino Hospital Credit Union.

My major goals for the coming year are:

- Expand training programs for staff nurses to increase awareness of budgets, etc.
- Enhance knowledge base in understanding of collective bargaining and political process from perspective of health care delivery.
- Ongoing orientation of new HNs and AHNs to budgets.
- Attendance at MOD Programs.

## NURSE RECRUITMENT AND EMPLOYEE RELATIONS COORDINATOR'S REPORT

I am responsible for the effective recruitment of qualified nursing personnel as well as for providing information and consultation to all individuals and groups in nursing service on any personnel relations matter.

My major achievments this year have been:

- Effective maintenance of total recruitment-retention program.
- Conduction of 456 pre-screening interviews, which resulted in the hiring of 129 total staff. The overall nursing turnover rate was 14.8%.

- Participation in ECH Critical Care Recruitment Committee.
- Conduction of first national recruitment trip for ECH. (Trip included interviewing in St. Louis, Boston, and New York City.)
- Participation in development of Bay Area Nurse Recruiter Association. Member of National Nurse Recruiters' Association.
- Development of overall recruitment and retention plan (long range).
- Coordinated and represented ECH nursing service at the annual S.F. Job Fair Oct. 1980, and at various high-school, college, and nursing-school and refresher-program career days.
- Developed a recruitment exhibit to be used at job fairs and career days.

My major goals for the coming year are:

- Participate in the formation of a hospital Recruitment and Retention Committee.
- Implement program for interval interviews on all RNs after 6 months of employment.
- Conduct exit interviews on all nurses resigning from ECH.
- Participate with Recruitment/Retention Committee to develop strategies aimed at reducing current vacancy rates.
- Participate in planning to incorporate greater numbers of new graduate nurses into ECH nursing service positions.

## INTERDEPARTMENT NURSING LIAISON COORDINATOR'S REPORT

I am responsible for establishing, updating, and monitoring nursing departmental policies and protocols and interdepartmental relationships.

My major achievements this year have been:

- Revision of nursing policy manual.
- Assisted with completion of exchange cart system on second floor.
- Assisted with policy development.
- Assisted with architectural planning and construction and decorating for nursing.
- Participated in the development of a nutrition committee.
- Participated in the implementation and evaluation of a nutritional pilot program.
- Participated in the development of a TPN Committee.
- Assisted with the implementation of new IV pumps.
- Assisted with nursing requests for capital purchases.
- Coauthored book on nursing decentralization.

My major goals for the coming year are:
- Revise and update nursing recovery room protocols.
- Develop nursing OR protocols.
- Assist with nourishment delivery system.
- Plan for replacement of gurneys and wheelchairs.
- Assist with reconstruction and redecorating of 2-East.
- Prepare for the Consolidated Accreditation and Licensure Survey.

## QUALITY ASSURANCE COORDINATOR'S REPORT

I am responsible for analyzing all patient cases that fall out as a result of generic screening criteria. I am responsible for maintaining a program that identifies the quality of nursing.

My major achievements this year have been:

- Provided concurrent monitoring of both nursing and medical staff performance.
- Assumed responsibility for seeing to it that fallouts were analyzed and remedial actions carried out.
- Contributed much to the education of nursing and medical staff in the early warning system and the audit process.
- Followed up on all nursing incident reports and provided feedback on a quarterly basis regarding trends.
- Coauthored an article on outcome charting, to be published in *Supervisor Nurse* in October 1981.
- Investigated all claims against hospital or MD.

My major goals for the coming year are:

- Establish a nursing concurrent review committee and develop purpose and objectives and evaluations.
- Update incident report matrices so that a mechanism for analysis of trends will be available.
- Become more invloved and provide direction for hospitalwide Q.A. program to meet JCAH standards.

## NURSING AUDIT COORDINATOR'S REPORT

I am responsible for maintaining a program that identifies and measures the quality of nursing care. I assist and relieve the quality assurance coordinator in analyzing all patient cases that fall out as a result of the early warning system.

My major achievements this year have been:

- Development with clinicians of the following:
    1. Revision of MSO concurrent audit tool.
    2. Revision of maternity and L&D concurrent audit tool.
    3. Concurrent audit tool for evaluating discharge planning.
    4. Retrospective audit criteria on 4–5 audits—findings reviewed with HNs and remedial action plans developed.
- Developed and implemented a system to give ancillary departments audit-result feedback specific to their department twice a year.
- Ongoing patient care survey via post-hospitalization questionnaires sent out to patients. Returned questionnaires were tallied and feedback given to staff.
- Assistance to quality assurance coordinator in reviewing quality care under the early warning system.
- Coaching and tracking of the audit process and the early warning system to nursing staff (ongoing process).

- Developed and implemented a remedial action form for concurrent audits.
- Participated in special retrospective audits.

My major goals for the coming year are:

- Act as a resource person to assist in the hospitalwide quality assurance program.
- Develop with assistance of clinicians concurrent audit tools for the elderly, alternate birth center, post partum, recovery room and pediatrics.
- Revise with assistance of clinicians, maternity tour questionnaire.
- Do a study on falls, and look at ways to lessen injuries.
- Implement and evaluate the Nursing Care Review Committee.
- Assist AKU in developing concurrent audit tool.

## REPORT OF THE NURSING COORDINATORS, 3-11 SHIFT

We are responsible for the administration of the hospital on the 3-11 shift. We are available as resources to assistant head nurses, head nurses, and staff to assist in the identification and solving of problems related to patient care, quality assurance, and management.

Major achievements this year have been:

- Assistance to nurse recruiter in recruitment activities.
- Participation in development of recruitment/retention plan for nursing service.
- Assistance to quality assurance in conducting audits on the 3-11 shift.
- Provision of emotional support to staff, patients, and relatives.
- Function as liaison between PRN and nursing administration.

Major goals for the coming year are:

- Participate in implementation of recruitment/retention plan.
- Increase knowledge base re marketing/recruitment/retention issues.

## REPORT OF THE NURSING COORDINATORS, 11-7 SHIFT

As nursing coordinators we assume overall responsibility for the hospital during the 11 p.m.–7 a.m. shift. We are available to assist the staff in the identification and solving of problems related to patient care, quality assurance, and management.

Our major achievements this year have been:

- Actualization of resource role in problem identification and problem solving on unit management and patient care issues.
- Reinstitution of regular AHN meetings.
- Participation in the preparation of statistical information for nursing unit daily productivity monitoring.
- Provision for emotional support to staff, patients, and relatives.
- Participation in the task force to develop policies regarding the planned and unplanned transfers to and from the critical care areas.

- Assistance to quality assurance in conducting nursing audits.
- Weekend and holiday staffing coordination for day shift.

Our major goals for the coming year are:

- To become more involved with staff development on night shift.
- To become involved in Nursing Care Review Committee.
- Continuation of the activities identified as achievements with focus on improving those supports when possible.
- Pursuit of continuing education programs.

## INFECTION CONTROL COORDINATOR'S REPORT

Infection control has several functions: (1) surveillance of community- and hospital-acquired infections; (2) consultation resource regarding isolation procedures and aseptic techniques; (3) provision of infection control related inservices; (4) participation in Infection Control and Product Evaluation and Safety Committees; (5) supervision/preparation of monthly infection statistical summaries for ECH and CDC; (6) reporting diseases/conditions to Board of Health.

The major achievements this year have been:

- Surveillance of community-acquired infections.
- Revising/updating isolation policy and procedure.

The major goals for the coming year are:

- Surveillance of community-acquired infections.
- Providing inservice programs on infection control for nursing and other departments.
- Preparing teaching module on isolation to be placed in the learning center.
- Revising/updating infection control manual of policies/procedures.
- Providing infection control information for orientation of new employees.
- Bulletin board—education/focal point for pertinent infection control data that could be utilized by staff.
- Participation in Infection Control and Product Evaluation and Safety Committees.
- Supervision/preparation of monthly infection control statistical summaries for ECH & CDC.
- Reporting diseases/conditions to Board of Health.

## DISCHARGE PLANNING COORDINATORS' REPORT

The discharge planning coordinators assist patients with complex post-hospitalization care needs by providing for appropriate and timely, continued care following their hospitalization, utilizing necessary in-house, community, and family resources.

The major achievements this year have been:

- Formal presentation given to medical staff on discharge planning, scope of services, and current legislation that requires discharge planning as an essential health care component.
- Both discharge planning coordinators have also given formal and informal presentations to nursing staff this year.
- We have been instrumental in formally organizing our own local Santa Clara County Discharge Planners Association, and this year have planned, organized, and hosted the first discharge planners' statewide convention. (This two-day workshop addressed several current issues regarding rehabilitation services and centers, new legislation regarding conservatorships, new and upcoming Medi-Cal regs., and quality assurance and how it impacts discharge planning. This workshop met criteria for continuing education.)
- Met with state senator to discuss long-term care issues and problem placements.
- Streamlined casefinding activities via utilization referral system.
- Successfully completed writing of our department's policies and procedures.
- Have developed a discharge planning questionnaire to be incorporated into a quality assurance program.
- Have received peer review (eval.) via questionnaire regarding discharge planning services (feedback from medical staff).
- Have worked closely with director of education for respiratory therapy department in setting up the comprehensive pulmonary program.

The major goals for the coming year are:

- Increase staff to meet the demands of increasing caseload.
- Provide privacy and adequate space for interviewing and counseling patients/families.
- Continue visitation of community agencies and skilled nursing facilities.
- Continue monthly meetings with Long-Term Care Committee and plan to work with state officials to streamline placement of heavy care patients.

# NURSING UNIT REVIEW

## EMERGENCY DEPARTMENT HEAD NURSE'S REPORT

The major achievements of the department this year have been:

- Implementation of primary-nurse asignment system.
- Implementation of triage nurse system.
- Refinement of patient charges based on categorization of nursing time.

The major goals of the department for the coming year are:

- Implementation of cart exchange system.
- Implementation of productivity based on patient categorization.
- Completion of emergency department core curriculum.

## INTENSIVE CARE UNIT HEAD NURSE'S REPORT

The major achievements of the unit this year have been:

- Participation in the development and implementation of critical care course.
- Eight ICU nurses attended and completed critical care course with preceptor program updated to facilitate ten-week orientation of critical-care course orientees.
- Several nurses completed course on I.A.B.P.
- Smooth transition of administrative staff in ICU.

The major goals of the unit for the coming year are:

- Forecast census.
- Develop pre-op teaching program.
- Continue advanced cardiac life support certification.
- Begin preceptor support group.
- Develop tool to forecast ICU curriculum.
- All staff update skills via core curriculum.
- Retain stable staff, all shifts, by creative staffing.

## CARDIAC CARE UNIT HEAD NURSE'S REPORT

The major achievements of the unit this year have been:

- Completed core curriculum for beginning-level CCU nursing practice.
- Developed performance review manual.
- Pioneered creative staffing patterns in an attempt to maintain quality care during staffing shortages.
- Maintained high productivity.
- Maintained high concurrent audit scores.
- Maintained an active role in the CPR committee in order to upgrade emergency services.
- Participated in the development and implementation of the new critical care course preparing 4 RNs for CCU nursing practice.
- Spearheaded cardiac rehabilitation committee providing consistency and quality in patient education.
- CCU staff 90% certified in ACLS.

The major goals of the unit for the coming year are:

- Develop a support group program for spouses of patients who have suffered MIs.
- Develop core curriculum for CCU nursing practice at intermediate and advanced levels.
- Develop and implement the exercise component to cardiac rehabilitation.
- Maintain high productivity and concurrent audit scores.
- Update our preceptor program in order to support development of new recruits to critical care.
- Implement the exchange cart system.

## TRANSITIONAL CARE UNIT HEAD NURSE'S REPORT

The major achievements of the unit this year have been:

- Implementation of charting by progress note and observation/assessment sheet.
- Utilization of computerized arrythmia detection as well as increased telemetry availability (16).
- ACLS certification increased to 88% of RN staff.
- Implementation of orientation as a competency-based program which precedes core curriculum.
- Development and initial implementation of TCU core curriculum.
- Completion of design portion of new unit.
- Implementation of charge nurse guidelines.
- Revision of monitor nurse/tech role incorporating guidelines format.
- Successful experience with San Jose State and De Anza Nursing seniors utilizing TCU as clinical area.
- Participation in the El Camino Hospital nutritional pilot program.
- Participation in the development and implementation of the critical care course now being offered at DeAnza College.

The major goals of the unit for the coming year are:

- Increase ACLS certification to 100%.
- Increase participation of staff in pursuit of core curriculum.
- Continue planning for new unit with target date of July 1981.
- Increase effectiveness of informal/formal Critical-Care Complex communication.
- Continue exploring utilization of new graduates.
- Continued participation in and support of The Cardiac Rehabilitation Program.
- Participate in planning for optimum utilization of 4-West.

## LABOR AND DELIVERY HEAD NURSE'S REPORT

The major achievements of the unit this year have been:

- Implementation of block scheduling of c/sections, inductions, and outpatient antepartum tests.
- Implementation of creative staffing, after analysis of work distribution.
- Improved productivity in spite of 13% increased patient census.

The major goals of the unit for the coming year are:

- Implement primary nurse concept for ABC patients.
- Implement criteria for care of high-risk obstetrical patients.
- Continue surgical scrub and circulating training so that at least 75% of all c/sections done in L&D are cared for by L&D staff.

## NURSERY HEAD NURSE'S REPORT

The major achievements of the unit this year have been:

- Development and implementation of new flow sheets (I+O/resp. care).
- Development and implementation of Dextrostix policy.
- Implementation of sibling visitation.
- Preparation of nursery core curriculum with staff development.
- Development and implementation of intensive training periods for newborn resuscitation.
- Renovation of nursery, especially construction of access doors between L&D and maternity recovery room.
- Development and implementation of infant auto-safety program, including availability of infant care seats through ECH.
- Acquisition and utilization of new cardio-respiratory monitors in special care area.
- Revision of phototherapy policy and procedure to increase unit cost-effectiveness.
- Revision of nursery policy and procedure manuals.
- Development and implementation of intubation practice sessions.

The major goals of the unit for the coming year are:

- Implement exchange cart system for supplies.
- Implement computer-assisted nursing care planning.
- Implement core curriculum.
- Implement teaching flow sheet.
- Revise labor standards.
- Continue to improve intracomplex working relationships.

## MATERNITY HEAD NURSE'S REPORT

The major achievements of the unit this year have been:

- Implementation of computer-assisted care planning.
- Development of core curriculum.
- Initiation of sibling visitation to further support our philosophy of family-centered care.
- Implementation and utilization by maternity and nursery staff of the maternity teaching progress record.
- Increased availability of flexible scheduling to meet the needs of the staff as well as those of the unit.

The major goals of the unit for the coming year are:

- Implement core curriculum for all new and existing employees on the maternity unit.
- Develop an audit tool for monitoring and documenting nursing care in the recovery room.
- Improved cohesiveness of the perinatal units through direct and honest communication.

## PEDIATRICS HEAD NURSE'S REPORT

The major achievements of the unit this year have been:

- Pediatrics has been caring for overflow maternity patients and providing rooming-in for those mothers who wish it.
- Increased numbers of parents staying with children.
- Microwave for patient and parent convenience.
- Have bulletin board exhibiting patients' artwork and community responses to the Pedi Tour.

The major goals of the unit for the coming year are:

- Question more sibling contact (aim for family unit cohesiveness).
- Decorating.

## 2-NORTH (SURGICAL) HEAD NURSE'S REPORT

During the past year 2-North has continued to care for surgical patients. The staff enjoys the mix of medical, surgical, and orthopedic patients which allows them to continually enhance their MSO skills.

The major achievements of the unit this year have been:

- Opened short-term surgical unit 12–14 beds on 2-West for 5 months.
- Ongoing updating in med-surg skills.
- Increased intershift communications through scheduled meetings.
- Participation of staff on all three shifts to effectively meet unit staffing needs with particular attention given to mix.

The major goals for the coming year are:

- Enhancement of discharge teaching.
- Enhancement of intershift participation.
- Responsible nurse concept adjusted to needs of RN on unit.
- Continued involvement of staff in management of unit.
- Involvement of each staff member in unit satisfaction and staff morale.

## 2-WEST (SURGICAL) HEAD NURSE'S REPORT

The major achievements of the unit this year have been:

- Achieved productivity goal.
- Improved quality and frequency of discharge teaching.
- Achieved established overall goal for concurrent audit review.
- Researched and developed an audio-visual preoperative teaching program which is being adapted for closed-circuit television.

The major goals of the unit for the coming year are:
- Improve documentation of discharge teaching records.
- Orient staff to preoperative teaching program.
- Achieve 90% score in all areas of patient care and care planning on concurrent audit reviews.

## 2-EAST (SURGICAL) HEAD NURSE'S REPORT

The major achievements of the unit this year have been:

- Maintenance of high quality nursing care.
- Maintenance of concurrent audit score of 90% or above.
- Formulation of active intershift council.
- Certification of majority of RNs in total parenteral nutrition protocol.
- Sustained active participation in several hospital committees by staff members.
- Development of charge nurse responsibilities (written).
- Development of resource nurse responsibilities (written).

The major goals of the unit for the coming year are:

- Continued high quality nursing care.
- Continued high level of staff satisfaction in nursing care

## 5-WEST (SURGICAL) HEAD NURSE'S REPORT

The major achievements of the unit this year have been:

- Certification of several staff nurses in CAPD.
- Implementation of flexible staffing plan.
- Development and implementation of monthly intershift meeting.
- Orientation of charge staff nurses to budget.

The major goals of the unit for the coming year are:

- Monthly peritoneal and hemodialysis inservice.
- Continue participation of all nurses in physical assessment classes.
- Enhancement of quality of patient discharge teaching.
- Certification of all RNs in CAPD.

## 5-EAST (ORTHOPEDIC) HEAD NURSE'S REPORT

The major achievements of the unit this year have been:

- Development of total-hip pre-op teaching program.
- Implementation of staff nurse intershift committee to problem solve intershift and unit issues.
- Development of orthopedic discharge teaching record.
- Implementation of 10-hour shift for most full-time employees.
- Increase staff involvement on nursing committees.
  Minimal staff shortages on any shift.

The major goals of the unit for the coming year are:

- Complete and implement pre-op teaching program for patients having total hip surgery.
- Implementation of orthopedic discharge teaching sheet.
- Remodel existing conference room on 5-East as a nurses' lounge.
- Increase unit educational programs.
- Increase retention of personnel.

## 6-WEST (MEDICAL) HEAD NURSE'S REPORT

The major achievements of the unit this year have been:

- Completion of the physical assessment class by the majority of the RN staff and participation in the hospital-based PA series by most of the remainder of the RN staff.
- Development and recent implementation of an orientation plan for unit charge nurses.
- Achievement of an overall productivity of 1.01 at the end of fiscal year '79–'80. (Our goal was .98.)
- Implementation of the medical teaching progress record.
- Increased participation by staff nurses in committees and as resource nurses.
- Harmonious working together of staff on all three shifts in the face of continued high patient acuity, loss of fellow staff, and position vacancies.

The major goals of the unit for the coming year are:

- Improvement in concurrent audit results by consistent achievement of 90% or above in all components—specifically aimed at the therapeutic and rehabilitative needs component of care planning.
- Increase the timely use of the medical teaching progress record.
- Development of a unit-level method of analyzing unit incident reports by shift for purposes of remedial action planning.
- Provision of unit inservice programs scheduled on a quarterly basis in the areas of pulmonary assessment and care, cancer/chemotherapy, diabetes, and hyperalimentation.
- Certification of a greater number of RN staff on all shifts in ABGs, hyperalimentation, and chemotherapy.
- Participation of selected charge nurses in budget and staffing workshops.
- Participation in a multi-disciplinary task force that addresses the issues of the hospitalization and post-hospitalization care needs of the elderly.
- Reseach feasibility of implementation of common progress note charting on 6-West.

## 6-EAST (MEDICAL) HEAD NURSE'S REPORT

The major achievements of the unit this year have been:

- Established 6-East orientation schedules by shifts for use of floats.

- Initiated intershift committee to problem solve and promote better communication with more staff involvement.
- Chemotherapy manual—learning module developed.
- Participated in development of refresher program.
- In-depth training of relief charge staff in management skills.
- Developed new procedure for gowning for isolation (all staff instructed).
- Clocks installed in all private rooms to provide better isolation techniques and promote better patient orientation.

The major goals for the coming year are:

- Chemotherapy certification for all staff administering chemotherapy.
- Better documentation of remedial action and follow-up on incident reports.
- Comfortable understanding of the Nurse Practice Act and its direct effect on staff practice (all RN staff).
- Complete body mechanics program—all staff.

# COMMITTEE AND TASK FORCE REVIEW

## CPR COMMITTEE CHAIRPERSON'S REPORT

The purpose of the multidisciplinary nursing CPR Committee is to standardize hospitalwide CPR training for hospital personnel (basic and advanced), to evaluate and recommend changes in equipment and techniques through review of CPR critiques and liaison with other departments and resources, and to monitor the standardization of all equipment on crash cart.

The major accomplishments of this committee have been:

- Reviewed all codes—followed up on problem areas.
- Designed a revised CPR record which was piloted on CCU and TCU and by 2-East nurses.
- Revised CPR Record on all crash carts 10/80.
- Med. module on crash carts was updated to include Bretyllium.
- CPR team roles changed—TCU now med. nurse; recorder assigned; massage—patient's own nurse.
- Pediatric CPR emergency protocol updated and flow chart developed for crash carts—both passed by Medical Executive Committee 10/80.

The major goals of this committee in the coming year are:

- Review codes in depth.
- Continue to address all problems related to hospital CPRs.

Committee Members:

- Seven nursing educators
- CCU staff nurse
- One physician
- Two pharmacists
- TCU head nurse
- ICU head nurse
  One respiratory therapist
- CCU head nurse

## DIABETIC RESOURCE COMMITTEE CHAIRPERSON'S REPORT

The purpose of this multidisciplinary committee is to develop, plan, and coordinate educational activities for patients/families with diabetes, to establish a model for evaluating diabetic education, to provide resource to nursing units for care of diabetic patients, to improve quality of diabetic care, and to provide skill training for staff in diabetic teaching.

The major accomplishments of this committee have been:

- Bimonthly dynamic presentations by staff nurses and patients on: "Sex and the Diabetic," "The Blind Diabetic," "Care of the Surgical Diabetic," and "Care of the Pregnant Diabetic."
- Diabetic manuals were updated to include the latest easy-to-use diabetic patient teaching materials.
- A 9-part module in the learning center for 10 hours of continuing education credit was developed to help new diabetic resource persons and others interested in diabetes become more skilled in diabetic patient teaching.
- Purchased "Sugar Babe" for patient teaching.
- Diabetic resource group sponsored a booth at El Camino Hospital Nursing's First Annual Sharing Night .

The major goals for this committee in the coming year are:

- Diabetic skills update workshop, Spring 1981
- Blood glucose monitoring in control of insulin dose in place of urine sugar testing—knowledge/skill meeting.
- Outpatient program development to include needs assessment of community program plan—implementation. Evaluation to follow in later months.

Committee Members:
- Two dietitians
- One occupational therapist
- Two pharmacists
- One assistant head nurse
- Twelve staff nurses

## MIS COMMITTEE CHAIRPERSON'S REPORT

The purpose of this committee is to provide input to proposed MIS system changes; to collect information, ideas, and suggestions regarding areas of development for MIS; and to problem solve with input of MIS problems.

The major accomplishments of this committee have been:

- Established that committee members have a basic knowledge of the MIS system and how it operates at El Camino Hospital.
- Identified problems, implemented solutions, and evaluated results on a multitude of MIS-related issues. These activities are followed on a process list, which is updated monthly.
- Participated in liaison with other departments in mutual problem solving.
- Established major communication link with units regarding MIS issues.

The major goals of this committee in the coming year are:

- Continued work on recommendations from nursing for MIS changes and on other issues brought to the committee regarding MIS.
- Maintain the strength of this committee.

Committee Members:

- 3-11 AHN or designated other from each unit
- MIS director
- MIS assistant director
- MIS staff RN
- Nursing audit coordinator—Q.A.
- One secretary

## NURSE PRACTICE COMMITTEE CHAIRPERSON'S REPORT

The function of the Nurse Practice Committee is to review, research, and make recommendations regarding issues impacting on the delivery of quality nursing services. This process usually results in development of procedures and protocols or referral to the Tripartite Committee for standardized procedures.

The major accomplishments of this committee have been:

- Many procedures and policies were developed and passed by the committee (examples: clinitest in presence of cephalosporins, chemotherapy, extubation, removal of pericardial catheter).
- Development of a process list to be used to follow issues/procedures that are presented.
- Program was presented to medical staff about nursing practice at El Camino Hospital.
- Information booth at nursing department's communication party.

The major goals for this committee in the coming year are:

- To familiarize administration, physicians, and nursing with Nurse Practice Committee.

    1. These groups channel appropriate requests through NPC.
    2. Nurses will be familiarized with the NPC through announcements of resolved issues in Nursing Newsletter.
    3. NPC will sponsor at least two activities relevant to nursing practice to increase committee visibility.

- To familiarize the NPC membership with nursing research.

    1. A program will be conducted for NPC on the research process.
    2. A system will be established for reviewing articles in *Nursing Research Journal*.
    3. Nurses will be invited to share their research activities.
    4. One researchable topic related to nursing practice at El Camino Hospital will be identified. This topic will be researched by a graduate student with support of the members of NPC.

Committee Members:

- Four nursing educators
- Two coordinators
- Director of nursing services
- Assistant director, MIS
- Five head nurses
- Three assistant head nurses
- Nine staff nurses

## NURSING CARE PLANNING COMMITTEE
## CHAIRPERSON'S REPORT

The function of this committee is to
develop and maintain a consistent/uniform care planning process,
clarify procedures for care planning,
standardize the application of care plans in charting,
identify areas in the care planning activity that need improvement,
review MIS matrices and recommend appropriate technologic changes,
increase communication regarding the care planning activity to others on the nursing unit, and
revise standard care plans.

The major accomplishments of this committee have been:

- Patient admission interview sheet.
- Assessment sheets—cardiovascular, respiratory, renal, abdominal.
- Revision of "common problems" in MIS.
- Development of audit tool to be used by staff nurses for unit QA audits.

The major goals of the committee in the coming year are:

- Revision of standard care plans.
- Development of standard care plans.

Committee Members:

- Fourteen staff nurses
- One head nurse
- One quality assurance coordinator
- One nursing educator
- MIS director
- MIS assistant director

## NURSING CARE REVIEW COMMITTEE'S REPORT

The Nursing Care Review Committee has just been formed. It will be a peer-review committee the purpose of which is to discuss and review serious nursing incidents. This in turn will benefit and educate the nursing staff. This committee will also have the responsibility for recommending action on issues requiring remedial action in order to maintain high quality patient care at El Camino Hospital.

The major goals for the coming year are:

- Review frequently occuring incidents.
- Review serious incidents.
- Recommend remedial action plans, feedback, and follow-up.
- Review charts from the Medical Concurrent Review Committee for appropriate nursing management.
- Summary of the cases reviewed and action taken will be reported to the Nursing Management Council on a quarterly basis by the committee chairperson.
- Develop a system for profiling patterns and trends.
- Develop a system to evaluate the success of the committee; such evaluation will be shared with nursing management council.

Committee Members:

- Two quality assurance coordinators
- Director of nursing services
- One nursing educator
- One nursing coordinator 11-7
- Two head nurses
- Two assistant head nurses
- Three staff nurses
- MIS director

## OSTOMY RESOURCE COMMITTEE CHAIRPERSONS' REPORT

The purpose of this committee is to provide quality ostomy patient care through use of resource nurses specially prepared to advise on up-to-date methods of appliance selection and skin-care programs and to provide for organized teaching of ostomy patients and families and ECH staff.

The major accomplishments of this committee have been:

- Update of the ostomy resource manual on each clinical unit.
- Audit of ostomy charts revealing an increase in quality of care given to ostomy patients at El Camino.
- Inservices for ostomy nurses.
- "Op-site for Decubitus Care."
- Reorganization of ostomy supplies for easy access in central service

The major goals of this committee in the coming year are:

- Quarterly inservice update to include Op-site for Decubitus Care, draining wounds.
- Proposal in beginning stages to evaluate need to train resource staff as E.T.

Committee Members:

- One head nurse
- Two assistant head nurses
- Four staff nurses

# PRODUCT EVALUATION COMMITTEE'S REPORT

The purpose of this committee is to evaluate new products and monitor the usage of nursing supplies with emphasis on quality of care and cost containment.

The major accomplishments of this committee have been:

- Recommended purchase of IV infusion pumps.
- Evaluation of items that projected a cost savings.

The major goals of this committee in the coming year are:

- Review of high-volume items and evaluation of those that indicate a cost savings.
- Standardization of items as much as possible.
- Increase nursing staff awareness of committee objectives.

Committee Members:

- Five staff nurses
- One head nurse
- Two nursing educators
- One nursing coordinator
- One materials manager
- One purchasing agent
- One bio-med engineer
- One management engineer
- Central distribution manager

# REACH-TO-RECOVERY RESOURCE COMMITTEE
# CHAIRPERSON'S REPORT

This committee's functions are to make available a copy of the Daisy folder to each mastectomy patient, to stimulate awareness and involvement in the Reach-to-Recovery program among members of the health team, to contact physicians to encourage Reach-to-Recovery referral, and to orient other nursing staff to Reach-to-Recovery.

The major accomplishments of this committee have been:

- We have provided Daisy informational folders to numerous breast-surgery patients.
- In addition, we have provided Reach-to-Recovery Rehabilitation kits to mastectomy patients, including exercise equipment, bra, foam filling, and literature with Reach-to-Recovery visitor.
- Breast examination module was developed for the learning center and successfully completed by 200 staff nurses.

The major goals of this committee in the coming year are:

- Daisy folder to each breast-surgery patient.
- Workshop on breast cancer: "New Management and Reconstructive Surgery".

Committee Members:

- Three staff nurses
- One head nurse

# Appendix H.  Glossary

**Accountability**
The responsibility and answerability for one's own actions.

**Accounting period**
The hospital's accounting system is based on 13 four-week accounting periods per year.

**Acuity**
A numerical measure of the care needed for an individual patient.

**Authority**
In decentralized nursing, the power to make necessary decisions about the patients for whom one is responsible and accountable.

**Autonomy**
The expectation that individual nurses will make their own decisions about patients instead of being required to seek permission or agreement from the next higher level of the nursing structure.

**Budgeted patient hours**
The number of hours expected to be used in patient care for the patient days forecast for a unit.

**Budget worksheet**
A sheet used to analyze productivity, the unit labor standard, and forecasted patient days in order to determine the staff needed for the coming budget period. The budget worksheet is extremely important to each unit because it serves as the basis by which they are able to hire staff for that period of time.

**Coaching**
The process of supporting growth and development in another.

**Complex**
A collection of units with common kinds of services and interests. For example, the Critical-Care complex is the combination of the Intensive Care, Coronary Care, Transitional Care, and Emergency units.

**Complex captain**
A head nurse either elected or selected ι serve as the coordinator, principally for communication, between the units in a complex and between complexes.

**Concurrent audit**
An assessment of the quality of patient care performed while the patient is still in the hospital.

**Contract**
An agreement between individuals that clarifies mutual responsibilities.

**Core staffing pattern**
A number arrived at by previous experience and information which indicates the number of full-time nurses that will be needed to care for the expected number of patients admitted to a given unit.

**Cost center**

A discrete reporting category that can be coded and used to isolate different functions within a nursing unit or department. Cost centers are used to identify and determine the distribution of time worked within a department.

**Criteria**

Criteria are the indicators used to measure the goals of patient care.

**Decentralization**

A way of organizing, communicating, and decision making that fosters autonomy, accountability, and authority at the practitioner level in nursing.

**Earned standard hours**

The number of hours "earned" is the labor standard times the unit of activity, such as patient days.

**Executive advisory committee**

A representative nursing group that meets at least once a month to discuss issues of interest to all nurses in the hospital and work on a chosen project.

**Expected (patient) outcomes**

Specific measurable behavior, knowledge, or clinical status of the patient that represents prevention, proper management, or resolution of a problem. Expected outcomes must be realistic, specific, directly observable, and measureable, and are the basis for charting patient progress.

**Feedback loop**

The loop that occurs when input into a system creates a reaction which returns to the source of the input.

**Full-time equivalent**

Each 80 hours per pay period means one full-time equivalent (FTE). The time, however, may be broken down into two half-time, four quarter-time or other variations, allowing for more flexibility in staffing. An FTE is the basis on which staffing is figured for budgeting purposes, even though the position may be filled by one or more persons.

**Head nurse**

A key figure in decentralization, the autonomous head of a nursing unit who plans his or her own budget, hires his or her own staff, is responsible for all the unit's patients, and is the cornerstone of care in the unit.

**Incident report**

A report of any accident or occurrence in which the hospital may be likely to incur liability because of action or lack of action.

**Labor analysis report**

A report that shows all the productive and nonproductive hours by job categories or paid time off for the total hospital.

**Labor distribution report**

The same information contained in the Labor Analysis Report, except that it indicates individuals by name rather than simply by job code. It provides the head nurse of the unit with the allocation of the time utilized every pay period.

**Labor performance report**
A summary of a unit's earned standard hours divided by the actual hours worked for all cost centers. It includes information about the unit's overall goal by pay period and year-to-date figures.

**Learning center**
A resource center established for staff's use on a 24-hour basis. Contains written modules for self-paced learning. Houses several types of audio-visual equipment and materials videocassettes, slide-sound programs, film strips, and audio tapes.

**Management Council**
A group from nursing service (mostly head nurses) that makes policy decisions, subject to approval of the director, and provides a means for communication.

**Medical information system (MIS)**
A hospitalwide system wherein a computer stores data and provides it, automatically or upon request, to the people who need to act upon it. The computer adds speed and accuracy to the transmission of information throughout the hospital and also performs many data-processing tasks such as sorting, copying, filing, summarizing, checking for abnormal data, charging, and a variety of other functions usually done by physicians, nurses, technologists, clerks, and other hospital personnel. A broad range of medical data (physicians' orders, test results, etc.) and administrative data (responsible party, insurance coverage, etc.) are processed by the computer.

**Nonproductive time**
Paid time off such as vacation, holiday, sick, or education leave.

**Nursing utilization**
The percentage figure obtained when required nursing hours are divided by the actual number of hours used in patient care.

**Paid time**
Any time for which an employee is paid. It includes both productive and nonproductive time.

**Patient dependency categorization report**
A summary of documented required hours for patient care divided by the actual hours worked in providing that care. In addition, the report also shows the acuity categories for all patients. The report is used to assist progress toward 100-percent utilization of the personnel in the unit. It is issued every two weeks through the hospital's management engineering department.

**Pay period**
A two-week period that corresponds to the time-card payroll period.

**Preceptors**
Staff nurses chosen for their clinical expertise and desire to teach, to act as buddies or guides for new employees during orientation.

**Primary care**
The concept that an individual nurse is entirely responsible for specific patient(s). Primary care seeks to personalize the relationship between patient and nurse and to involve them both in a cooperative effort at recovery of health. Primary care begins with the patient's admission to a unit and continues throughout his or her stay (and sometimes beyond discharge).

**Productive time**
Paid time spent at work in patient care, administrative functions, committee work, etc.

**Productivity goal**
A productivity index set as the goal for the coming year.

**Quality assurance**
The ongoing assessment of the quality of care rendered in the hospital. Its aim is to ensure that high-quality care can be rendered uniformly and consistently throughout the hospital.

**Quality assurance audit**
A method of determining the level of quality of care being rendered by a unit, an individual, or the hospital. Audits may be concurrent or retrospective and are central to the operation of any quality assurance program.

**Required nursing hours**
The amount of nursing care required to care for patients based on the patient categorization (assigned acuity).

**Resource nurse**
A staff nurse with specialized knowledge or skill in such areas as hyperalimentation, arterial blood gases, diabetes, ostomy, or cannula care. He or she is available to assist patients and nursing staff.

**Retrospective audit**
An assessment of the quality of care received during hospitalization but performed after the patient has been discharged from the hospital.

**Staffing board**
A large board displayed in the nursing office. It lists all nursing personnel by shift, name, special skill, unit, and status.

**Standard nursing care plan**
A care plan that is developed and prewritten as a guide for use with patients who experience "usual" problems.

**Work agreement**
An agreement between head nurse and a staff nurse both for specific working conditions (shift, etc.) and for a commitment to a term of employment, usually at least one year.

# Index